Edward Gutmann

The Watering Places and Mineral Springs of Germany, Austria and Switzerland

with notes on climatic resorts and consumption, sanitariums, peat, mud, and sand baths, whey and grape cures

Edward Gutmann

The Watering Places and Mineral Springs of Germany, Austria and Switzerland
with notes on climatic resorts and consumption, sanitariums, peat, mud, and sand baths, whey and grape cures

ISBN/EAN: 9783337198299

Printed in Europe, USA, Canada, Australia, Japan

Cover: Foto ©Andreas Hilbeck / pixelio.de

More available books at **www.hansebooks.com**

BADEN-BADEN.

THE WATERING PLACES AND MINERAL SPRINGS

OF

GERMANY, AUSTRIA, AND SWITZERLAND;

WITH

NOTES ON CLIMATIC RESORTS AND CONSUMPTION, SANITARIUMS, PEAT, MUD, AND SAND BATHS, WHEY AND GRAPE CURES, &c.

A POPULAR MEDICAL GUIDE.

BY

EDWARD GUTMANN, M. D.

With Illustrations, Comparative Tables, and a Colored Map, explaining the Situation and Chemical Composition of the Spas.

New York:
D. APPLETON AND COMPANY,
1, 3. AND 5 BOND STREET.
1880.

COPYRIGHT BY
D. APPLETON AND COMPANY.
1880.

⁎ *The author would be much obliged for any corrections or suggestions, which can be sent to his residence, 120 East 58th Street, New York City.*

PREFACE.

From year to year the stream of English and Americans travelling to the Continent is increasing; of these, quite a considerable number afflicted with the various ailments which overwhelm suffering humanity, visit the various watering places of Central Europe. Unacquainted with the continental mode of living, they feel themselves uncomfortable during the greater part of their sojourn.

For such I intend to write a little book—not a learned discourse on the physiological effects or chemical compositions of the springs, but a POPULAR MEDICAL GUIDE, for the purpose of making them familiar with the arrangements, manners, and customs of living, at the *principal* watering places of Central Europe. Of these I shall give a brief description, with notes on the shortest routes of access. I shall also enumerate some general rules for the use of mineral waters, whose chemical constituents and medical application will be sufficiently explained to enable the reader to obtain a general knowledge of their efficacy.

However, I beg leave to remark, that every patient who intends to visit a watering place should not do so without having consulted an experienced physician, in order to ascertain which spring he should resort to, as it often happens that patients arriving at a spring not suited for their particular case are sent away to another, often far-distant, watering place.

Having for the last ten years frequented all the important watering places of Germany, Austria, and Switzerland, partly as a patient, partly for the purpose of obtaining a thorough knowledge of the same, I venture to compose, and present to the travelling public, this little guide-book.

A few notes on *climatic health resorts* will be annexed, which may prove useful to those patients who have a dislike to the use of mineral waters, and are desirous of obtaining a general recreation by means of mountain or sea-air, bodily exercise, and suitable diet.

A map showing the position of the principal springs will be added.

Quite a number of excellent works on balneology have been of great service to me; I mention Helft's, Braun's, and Kisch's "Balneotherapie;" Lersch's

"Fundamente der practischen Balneologie;" Beneke's "Balneologische Briefe;" and especially Dr. Th. Valentiner's "Balneotherapie" (1876); the last-named a very elaborate work, containing treatises on the various mineral waters, composed by Dr. Valentiner and other experienced bath physicians.[1]

Besides these works, a large number of monographs on various baths, and several guide-books, especially Baedeker's, have been consulted with great benefit.

I am also indebted to Professor Beneke of Nauheim, Dr. Lersch of Aachen, Dr. Gans, senior, of Karlsbad, Dr. Schreiber of Aussee, Dr. Röhrig of Wildungen, and to many other colleagues, for the valuable information I received from them on my tours through the various watering places.

THE AUTHOR.

LONDON, *November*, 1879.

---

[1] It has been deemed expedient to retain such expressions as bath physician, bath cure, bath rule, &c., as better expressing the meaning of the German words *Bade-Arzt, Bade-Kur, Bade-Regel*, than their English synonyms.

CONTENTS.

Part I.

GENERAL REMARKS ON WATERING PLACES AND THE USE OF MINERAL WATERS.

CHAPTER I.

ON THE BENEFIT OF VISITING WATERING PLACES.

	PAGE
Who should travel—Benefit of travelling to patients—Change of air, and of living—Imported mineral waters	1

CHAPTER II.

PREPARING FOR THE JOURNEY.

Selection of a spa—Who should not travel—The best time for a bath course	6

CHAPTER III.

THE TRIP TO THE CONTINENT.

(1) From London—(2) From New York—Money—Language—Passport—Lodgings—Bath physicians	9

CHAPTER IV.

GENERAL FEATURES OF THE CONTINENTAL WATERING PLACES.

The conversation-house — Kurgarten — Promenades — Hotels — Society — Morality — Bazaar — Cure-tax — Prices for baths 15

CHAPTER V.

BATH LIFE AND BATH RULES.

A general rule—Morning scenes at the fountain—How to drink—How much to drink—The morning coffee and coffee gardens—Clothing—*Tables d'hôte*—Sleep—Active exercise—Concerts—Mental labour—Theatre—Dancing—Company—Time for bathing—Temperature—Duration and number of baths—Badfriesel . 23

CHAPTER VI.

THE DIET DURING THE BATH CURE.

Importance of the diet—General rules—What patients may eat and drink—Beer—Preparatory course—After-cure—After-effects—Sight-seeing 42

CHAPTER VII.

WATER AND AIR.

Internal use of water—Absorption—Cold water—Warm water—Mineral water—External use of water—Cold, hot, and indifferent baths—Mineral-water baths—Absorption by the skin—City, country, mountain, and sea air 53

CONTENTS. ix

Part II.
TOPOGRAPHICAL REVIEW OF THE WATERING PLACES.

PAGE

Introductory remarks—The places which will be described
—Hotels—Physicians 64

CHAPTER I.
THE WATERING PLACES OF GERMANY.

I. Northern Germany: Nenndorf, Eilsen, Rehme, *Pyrmont*, Meinberg, Lippspringe, Inselbad, Driburg . 68
II. Western and Middle Germany: *Aachen* (Aix-la-Chapelle), Burtscheid, Neuenahr, Bertrich, *Kreuznach*, Münster-am-Stein, *Wiesbaden*, Langenschwalbach, Schlangenbad, *Ems*, Weilbach, Soden, *Homburg*, Nauheim, *Kissingen*, Bocklet, Brückenau, Wildungen 75
III. Southern Germany: *Baden-Baden*, Wildbad, Cannstadt, Reichenhall, Kreuth 102
IV. Eastern Germany: Obersalzbrunn, Warmbrunn, Landeck, Reinerz, Cudowa 113
Appendix:—Hotels in Bremen, Hamburg, Cologne, Munich, Frankfort, Dresden, Berlin 117

CHAPTER II.
THE WATERING PLACES OF AUSTRIA.

I. The Bohemian spas: *Karlsbad*, Teplitz, *Marienbad*, Franzensbad, Elster, Johannisbad 121
II. The spas in Middle Austria: Baden, Vöslau, Hall, *Ischl*, Aussee, Gastein 146
III. The spas in Southern Austria: Gleichenberg, Tobelbad, oRitsch, Neuhaus, Tüffer, Römerbad, Villach, spas in Tyrol, Innischen 154

CHAPTER III.

THE WATERING PLACES OF SWITZERLAND.

Baden — *Ragatz-Pfäffers* — Alveneu — *St. Moritz* — Le Prese—Bormio—Tarasp—Leuk 162

Part III.

CHEMICAL COMPOSITION AND THERAPEUTICAL APPLICATION OF THE MINERAL WATERS.

General remarks—Classification 174

CHAPTER I.

ALKALINE WATERS.

Soda—Carbonic acid—Glaubersalt—Simple alkaline waters—Alkaline muriated—Alkaline saline waters—Ems, Karlsbad, Marienbad, &c. . . . 176

CHAPTER II.

SALINE WATERS.

Saline springs—Chloride of sodium—Saline Baths—Soolbäder—Carbonic acid—Thermal saline baths—Baden-Baden, Kissingen, Wiesbaden, &c. 198

CHAPTER III.

SULPHUR WATERS.

General remarks—Sulphuretted hydrogen—Cold sulphur waters—Warm sulphur waters—Aachen, Neundorf, &c. 218

CHAPTER IV.

IRON WATERS.

Internal use of iron and iron water—Iron baths—Absorption of the iron—Pyrmont—St. Moritz—Langenschwalbach, &c. 227

CHAPTER V.

EARTHY WATERS.

Definition—Carbonate of lime—Sulphate of lime—Wildungen—Leuk, &c. 239

CHAPTER VI.

INDIFFERENT THERMAL WATERS.

Definition—Nerve baths—Effects of the baths—Indications—Teplitz—Gastein—Ragatz, &c. . . . 245

Part IV.

CLIMATOLOGICAL AND BALNEOLOGICAL NOTES.

CHAPTER I.

CLIMATIC HEALTH-RESORTS, WITH SPECIAL REFERENCE TO PULMONARY CONSUMPTION.

On consumption—Alpine heights—Change of air—Rules for patients travelling south—Warm air—Equability of air—Sunshine—Health-resorts, and intermediate stations—Clothing—Diet of consumptives—Sight-seeing—Occupation—Madeira—*Cairo*—Palermo—Cata-

	PAGE
nia—Ajaccio—Hyères—Cannes—*Nice*—Mentone—San Remo—Rome—Naples—Venice—Meran—Bozen—Gries—Arco—Montreux—Vevey—Clarens—Elevated regions—Sanitariums—Görbersdorf—Davos—Summer resorts—Seaside resorts—Ostend—Scheveningen—Norderney—Borkum—Sylt—Heligoland	253

CHAPTER II.

MISCELLANEOUS CURES.

Peat, mud, sand, pine-needle, and herb baths—Milk, whey, kumys, and grape cures—Herb juices—Hydropathic treatment 286

CHAPTER III.

THERAPEUTICAL RECAPITULATION.

Diseases of the digestive and respiratory organs; of the urinary and uterine system; of the skin; and of the nervous system—Constitutional diseases . . . 301

APPENDIX.

Comparative Tables of the principal mineral constituents
of the mineral waters 318
Coin Table 326

INDEX OF WATERING PLACES AND HEALTH-RESORTS . 327
GENERAL INDEX 329

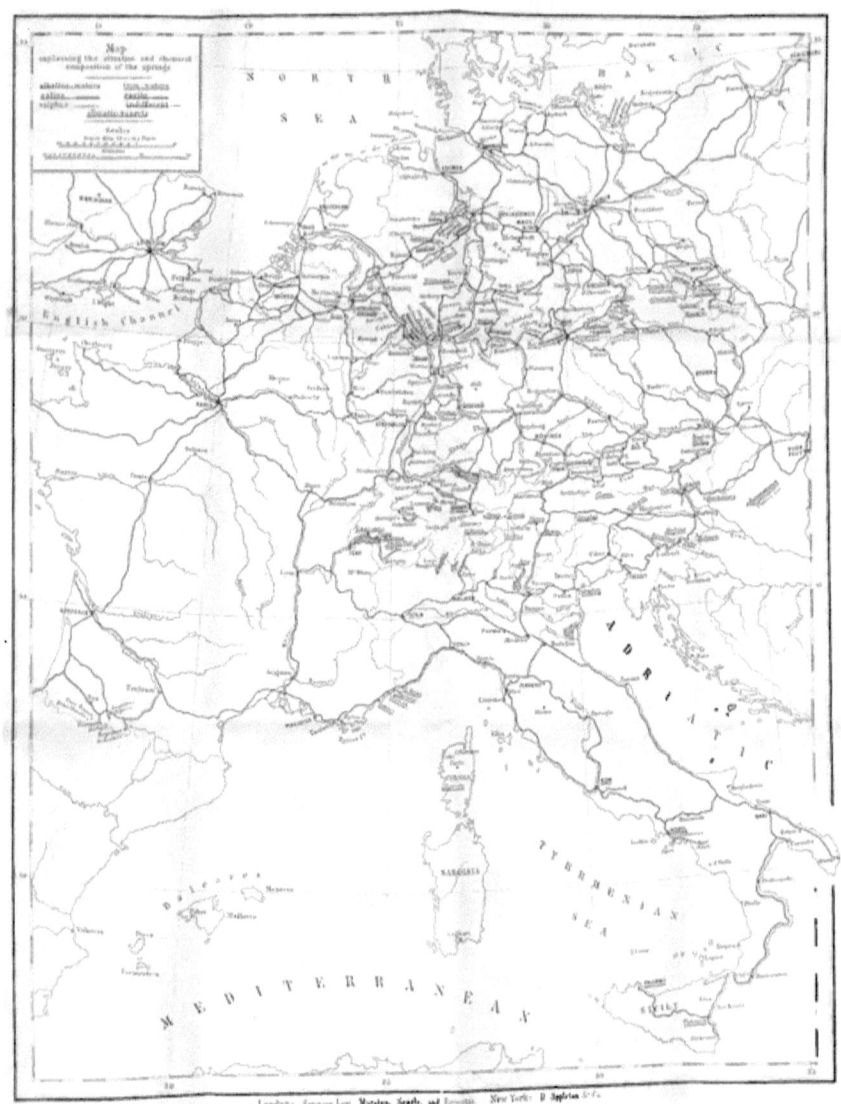

THE
Watering Places and Mineral Springs
OF
GERMANY, AUSTRIA, AND SWITZERLAND.

PART I.

GENERAL REMARKS ON WATERING PLACES AND THE USE OF MINERAL WATERS.

" Mens sana in corpore sano."

CHAPTER I.

ON THE BENEFIT OF VISITING WATERING PLACES.

THE English and Americans are travelling nations. It is the old restless spirit of wandering which inspires them—the same spirit which impelled the Teutonic tribes to overrun the Roman Empire, and which once drove the Anglo-Saxons from their seat in the northern part of Germany to England, and the English to America and all the other portions of the globe. This spirit is revived every spring, when nature awakens, and inspires all living beings with fresh energy. It is then that the hearty sons of Old

England gird their loins and cross the Channel by thousands, and the fair daughters of America crowd the swift ocean steamer on their European tour.

A trip to the continent is nowadays an indispensable requisite to the so-called fashionable world, and in this case all joyfully submit to the easy yoke of that pitiless queen called *fashion*. Happily, this fashion need not fear the verdict of the most scrupulous moralist, for travelling is a useful and wholesome practice; and although the great mass of travellers undoubtedly undertake the voyage *only* for the sake of pleasure, there are, nevertheless, a great many who are impelled by the desire to obtain a thorough knowledge of the customs and habits, arts and sciences, of the continental nations. And there are many others, whose mind and body are so overworked by the cares and troubles of business life, which puts such an enormous strain on the mental capacity, that a trip across the water is not only a much needed relaxation, but often an indispensable remedy to restore their health. Moreover, the sojourn in a climatic health-resort, situated in a mountainous region several thousand feet above the sea, proves highly efficacious to invigorate and strengthen a shattered constitution. These climatic resorts are very numerous in the Alpine regions of Central Europe, in Switzerland, Tyrol, Styria, &c. Here we find sanitariums fitted up in the most elaborate and practical style, with the best accommodation for patients, and under the supervision of experienced physicians. Americans, especially, are obliged to resort to these

European places, as America has no regular sanitariums.

Professor Loomis, of New York, in a lecture before the American Medical Association, delivered, in Buffalo, in June, 1878, has very properly and urgently recommended the erection of sanitariums. "It seems to me," he said, "that the necessities of our time are demanding the establishment not only of well-organized and thoroughly equipped sanitariums by the sea, in the mountains, in the cold regions of the north, and in the warm regions of the south, but that our mineral springs should be utilized for the cure of disease." (*Medical Record*, 1879.) This will be, for some time to come, a *desideratum*, and American patients are obliged to go abroad in search of sanitariums.

Finally, a large number of travellers are patients, who undergo the hardships of the voyage for the sole purpose of regaining their health by the use of a continental spa. Many efficacious waters—as, for instance, those of Karlsbad, Marienbad, Kissingen, &c.—are not equalled either in England or in America. The latter has a multitude of mineral springs in all parts of the wide country, but many of these are scarcely known, or have not been accurately analyzed, or are difficult of access. At all events, a visit to a *foreign* spa has some advantages, which cannot always be attained at home. The voyage in itself is generally exceedingly beneficial to many patients, especially to those affected with disorders of the abdominal organs, or with nervous affections resulting therefrom.

A protracted sea voyage, as it is undertaken by those who cross the ocean, is even far more beneficial, particularly to invalids whose constitution is impaired by diseases of long standing. The fresh sea-air, free from organic impurities, impregnated with salt, and rich in ozone, is invigorating and strengthening; it increases the appetite, promotes the digestion, and improves the assimilation and nutrition. Therefore Celsus already has recommended long sea voyages to patients affected with bronchial catarrhs, consumption, &c.

Of no less importance is the entire change in the mode of *living*, and the different kinds of society which English and Americans meet on the continent. To these, everything there is new; food, company, climate, hotels, all differ from what they are accustomed to see at home. The enforced alteration of diet and habits, the giving up of a long practised routine of daily life, the ease and comfort enjoyed by the temporary discontinuance of business, all this is eminently beneficial to a patient; and as most of the watering-places are situated in picturesque and pleasant regions, surrounded by forests or mountains, the novelty of scenery, the fresh, bracing mountain air, the daily exercise, are powerful agents in perfecting a cure.

In fact, all persons afflicted with *chronic* diseases, which are curable and proper objects for a treatment by mineral waters, should resort for a short time to a mineral spring, not only on account of its curative powers, but even more for the sake of relaxation, of fresh, pure air, and proper, wholesome diet.

Natural mineral waters, securely bottled, being nowadays exported to all parts of the globe, many believe them to be fully as efficient when taken at the patient's residence, as when drunk at the spring. This I believe to be a mistake. A regular strict treatment, as it is enforced by the physicians of a well regulated watering place, cannot be carried on at home. Business, family, old habits of living, and more often, divers irregularities of living, prevent the patient from adhering strictly to the rules prescribed for the use of the waters; he would not rise early in the morning for the sake of drinking a few glasses of water; afraid of neglecting his business, he would not spend several hours of the day for necessary exercise; nor would he wish to have the diet of the whole family changed on his account, because the usual diet does not agree with the mineral water, and so on. Moreover, there are waters whose efficacy mainly depends on their high natural temperature: it would hardly be possible for any patient, however careful, to raise the heat of the bottled water every morning to exactly the same degree. Other springs, particularly those impregnated with carbonic acid, lose that natural, fresh, prickling taste, which makes them so agreeable when taken on the spot, and which contributes a good deal to their universal popularity.

CHAPTER II.

PREPARING FOR THE JOURNEY.

THE first question to be settled is : which bath shall be visited by the invalid. This must be decided by the physician after careful examination, the patient himself, even with the aid of the best work on balneology, not being able to make the proper selection. It requires not only a full understanding of the particular case on the part of the examining physician, but also a thorough knowledge of the chemical constituents and medicinal effects, the climate, arrangements, locality, and even society of the various watering places. Some patients, having a predilection for elegant, fashionable society, would prefer to visit one of the fashionable luxurious, expensive spas near the Rhine ; while others would feel far more comfortable, and would derive more benefit, by resorting to one of the quiet, secluded, and cheaper, but not less efficient baths in Styria or Silesia. English and Americans, on account of the shorter route, may rather select a spa in the western part of Germany than one in Bohemia, if the same effect can there be obtained. A mountain climate at an elevation of 4000 feet above the sea might be very wholesome to some patients affected with bronchial catarrhs, while to others, suffering from the same malady, it would be deleterious. These and many other circumstances must be considered by a conscientious physician when selecting a bath for his patient.

And here I believe it opportune to remark, that patients in the last stages of consumption, or Bright's disease, or other chronic affections, should not be allowed to undergo the hardships and the excitement of a trip to a watering-place, thereby sacrificing the little amount of strength they still possess, for the imaginary hope of an impossible cure. It is the sacred duty of a physician to dissuade them from the journey; though very often the contrary takes place. Every bath physician during the bath season, has the opportunity of examining quite a number of incurable invalids, who have been sent to the spa by unscrupulous medical advisers, never again to return to their homes. Far away from their families, surrounded by strangers, more helpless and suffering than ever so before, they vainly long for the tender care of their relatives during the last days of their earthly pilgrimage.

In order to save the bath physician time and trouble, every invalid should hand him a certificate from his usual attending physician, briefly stating the history and nature of his case.

The best seasons for a bath cure are the spring and summer, the time from the first of May until the middle of September being the most favourable on the continent in regard to weather and temperature. Americans should depart in April, in order to commence the cure early in spring, particularly if, as is usually the case, they desire to travel when having terminated the bath course.

German poets are very enthusiastic in praise of spring, and undoubtedly it is the most delightful season of the year on the continent.

Every one knows the influence of the weather on the disposition; invalids are even far more affected by it: they feel better and more cheerful when the sun shines warm and bright; they are depressed and desponding when clouds darken the sky. Therefore it is not surprising that all writers on balneology recommend the beginning of a bath-cure when nature awakens from the long sleep of winter, the blossoms of trees and plants shoot forth, and new life is infused to all creation. Constant exercise in the open air being essential for the success of the treatment, it is obvious that this can be best attained during the fine spring and summer months.

Hot mineral waters, which produce easy perspiration, and sometimes congestions of the brain, should be taken during the cooler days of spring; it is also advisable for irritable, nervous persons, and for those with an apoplectic habit and a strong disposition to perspire, to commence treatment early in the spring. Old invalids, convalescents after severe diseases, and rheumatic patients, may rather defer their bath-course to the warm summer days, being then in less danger of taking cold. Iron waters and cold mineral waters are generally better tolerated during the summer season.

CHAPTER III.

THE TRIP TO THE CONTINENT.

I. *From London to the Continent.*

THE most favoured routes between London and the continent are—

 (*a*) From Dover to Calais, twice a day in 1¾ hours (Railway from London to Dover in 2 to 4 hours).

 (*b*) From Dover to Ostend twice a day, but once only on Saturdays and Sundays, in 4 to 5 hours.

 (*c*) From Harwich to Rotterdam, daily, in 13 hours (Railway from London to Harwich in 2 to 3 hours).

 (*d*) From Queenborough to Flushing every evening (Sundays excepted), in 9 to 10 hours (Railway from London to Queenborough in 2 hours).

 (*e*) From London to Bremen, twice a week, in 36 hours.

 (*f*) From London to Hamburg, five times a week, in 40 hours.

II. *From New York to the Continent.*

There are three lines of steamers sailing from New

York *directly to the continent*, which are particularly patronized by American travellers. These are—

(*a*) The North German Lloyd steamers leave New York for *Bremen* every Saturday at 3 p.m. (landing passengers at Southampton).

(*b*) The Hamburg-American Steamship Company steamer leaves New York every Thursday at 3 p.m. for *Hamburg* (landing passengers at Plymouth and Cherbourg).

(*c*) The General Transatlantic Company's steamers leave New York every Wednesday for *Havre*.

All the steamers of these lines have first class accommodations and moderate prices, a reduction being allowed for return tickets. The second and third lines are convenient for passengers desirous of visiting Paris, before going to a watering-place; those wishing to go directly to Germany should take the Bremen or Hamburg line.

Landed on *terra firma*, the patient should travel slowly, and by short distances, to the place of destination, especially avoiding night travel; for should he arrive fatigued and exhausted, he would be unable for some time to commence the course. Railway travelling on the continent is generally not very comfortable, the railway carriages on most of the roads being divided into small compartments, with deficient ventilation, bad air, and without any of the accommodations with which, for instance, the railway-carriages on the American roads are provided.

Most earnestly I would advise English and Americans who are about to visit the spas of Central Europe, viz.: of Germany, Austria, and Switzerland, to study the German language before their departure; a little knowledge will be very useful, because those entirely ignorant of it are subject to a great deal of annoyance and loss of money. English, and even more Americans, when travelling on the continent are generally overcharged; of the latter each one is considered a Crœsus. And this indeed is not surprising, as many who had become rich during the war and the greenback millennium rushed to Europe, and squandered the money in a most extravagant, and often ridiculous manner. And our German and Swiss friends were not slow to take advantage of this circumstance. It has often happened that Americans not acquainted with the German money and language, when asked for payment in cafés or restaurants, would hand their pocket-books to the waiters for the purpose of taking out the required sum. Such a confidence in the honesty of waiters, servants, or even proprietors of public places or shops, is entirely out of place; most of them are unscrupulous persons, who take every possible advantage of the ignorance of strangers.

My advice, based on the experience of many years' travelling, is: not to trust such persons at all, but to scrutinize carefully every bill of charge, *especially if presented by hotel-keepers shortly before leaving*.

The coin used in France and Switzerland is the *franc* (1 franc = 100 centimes) = $9\frac{1}{2}$ pence English and 19 cents. American money; the legal coin of Germany is the *mark* (1 Mark = 100 Pfennige) = 1 shilling English and 24 cents American money. Austria has the *florin* or *Gulden* (1 fl. = 100 Kreutzers) equal to 2 shillings or 49 cents. It is always profitable to be provided with some foreign money, in order to defray the necessary expenses when landing on foreign soil.

I call the attention of all who have never travelled on the continent to the fact, that charges for baggage are very high on all continental railways; only 50 lbs. are allowed to be carried free of charge, and even this privilege is not granted on all roads. Every trunk is carefully weighed at the station, and every pound must be paid for. Ladies who are in the habit of taking a large number of good, solid, heavy trunks with them, may take notice of this rule, if desirous of saving much money. The freight charges are lower if the trunks are sent by freight-trains (*Eilgut*), but they often arrive far later than their owner at the place of destination. Gentlemen fond of *good* cigars should supply themselves, but not with too large a quantity, because they are obliged to pay duty on them on the frontier of every country through which they pass, this being the only dutiable article for which the custom-house officers are on the constant lookout. A small quantity is allowed to pass free of duty.

It is a good precaution to procure a passport from the government before leaving home: the continental governments, in consequence of the recent attempts on the life of several sovereigns, are anxiously controlling the travelling public, and in some places—as in Berlin—the passport of every stranger must be delivered to the hotel keeper, in order to be examined by the police—an annoyance which had been abolished for a very long time. Americans are rarely molested in Europe; but being unacquainted with the laws and regulations, they may possibly become involved in difficulties with the authorities; in this case a passport will prove their identity, and save them a good deal of trouble.

Having arrived at the watering place, the best one can do is to settle for some time by hiring a furnished room. To live in hotels is not customary on the continent, except for a short stay.; and patients particularly, who always require rest, should never remain long in noisy hotels. The rooms selected should be high and airy, and if possible with a southern exposure, and not far from the spring; for it is very unpleasant, particularly on rainy days, to be obliged to march a long distance to the spring early in the morning, and to commence drinking when more or less fatigued or overheated.

After a protracted journey the patient should not hurry to begin the cure at once, but should rather rest a day or two, in order to recreate and regain his full strength. The next important step to be taken is, to consult an experienced bath physician. To enter upon a bath-course without medical advice would not be prudent; bath physicians know best the operations of the springs. Being in the habit of attending for years to a large number of patients suffering with similar affections, they acquire a thorough knowledge of these, and quite a routine in their treatment. It cannot be denied that it is precisely this routine which often induces them to treat the patients in a certain uniform manner, and great complaints on this matter are heard at every watering place; but in spite of this, no patient should neglect to seek the advice of a bath doctor. Of course, there are many who believe that mineral water, being indifferent medicine, can be taken *ad libitum*, and without any detriment; but this is a great mistake; many springs are powerful remedies, and when indiscriminately used, have often proved dangerous to patients. Others, seeing no immediate result of the treatment, travel from one spring to another. This is unreasonable. Give the spring you have selected a fair trial; do not expect to be cured within the short time of a few weeks, of a chronic disease of long standing; *do not become impatient; remain, drink, bathe, and you will succeed.*

CHAPTER IV.

GENERAL FEATURES OF THE CONTINENTAL WATERING PLACES.

A CERTAIN uniformity of the institutions exists at most of the watering places of Central Europe. The experience and practice of many years have demonstrated what arrangements are necessary for the comfort and entertainment of the visitors; thus they are mostly alike, the requirements of the patients being almost the same at the various spas. Everywhere do the authorities rival each other in their efforts to make their respective places as attractive as possible, in order to gain the most extensive patronage, as the welfare of their inhabitants mainly depends on their earnings during the bath season. A great difference exists in the magnificence and magnitude of the establishments. Of course they are more extensive and more elegant at the fashionable and renowned spas, as for instance Karlsbad or Wiesbaden, than at the quiet modest, unpretending places of the Black Forest or Switzerland. The centre of attraction in nearly all of them, is the *conversation-house*, or *Kurhaus;* here the visitors flock together during certain hours of the day, either for the purpose of drinking or bathing—as in many spas the springs and bathing-rooms are in it or near by—or for entertainment. It always contains a large concert and ball-room, handsomely, and in some of the fashionable Rhenish baths, as in Homburg and Baden-Baden, even extravagantly fitted up, elegant dining-rooms, billiard-rooms, and comfortable reading-rooms, provided with a multitude of the principal English, French, and German newspapers and periodicals. The restaurants connected with the conversation-houses are generally first class in price and quality.

Adjoining the *Kurhaus* is generally the *Kurgarten*, the pride of every well-organized watering place, with large trees hundreds of years old, whose shade affords ease and comfort to the patients, while drinking, promenading, or listening to the music. Here every morning from six to eight o'clock, a band under the leadership of an experienced conductor, performs select compositions of the best masters. In the afternoon and evening, concerts given at the *Kurgarten*, or sometimes at other public places, also attract the majority of visitors. To spend several hours of the day in the garden, inhaling the fresh pure air, listening to the masterpieces of Mozart, Beethoven, Weber, etc., chatting, gossiping, and drinking excellent coffee, is considered the greatest charm of bath life. Balls are also arranged. Those fond of the theatre or the opera have the opportunity of hearing celebrated actors and singers, who, during the bath season, travel from one fashionable place to another, winning laurels and money.[1]

[1] Most of the watering places have an English church, where the usual services are held.

Shady promenades, and walks through the forests, kept in good order and provided with many resting-places, encourage the patients to stroll about even during the hottest hours of the warm summer days. This is of the greatest importance, as constant though moderate exercise is absolutely necessary for the success of the treatment. For the same reason excursions on a small scale are highly recommendable, so much the more as the scenery around most of the springs is generally picturesque and interesting. Those who wish to derive the most benefit, may walk ; invalids too weak to walk for any length of time, may ride on mules or in carriages. Little waggons drawn by donkeys can be hired for a moderate charge by the hour or day. Wherever you go or drive you find cafés and restaurants, where coffee, milk, seltzer water, and other refreshments are served at fair prices. Nowhere are you in danger of being molested or insulted by rude people ; a vigilant and attentive police guard your personal security.

The hotels vary in size and comfort according to the class of customers they receive. Some, having the reputation of being patronized by the high nobility, or the high functionaries of state, or the nabobs of the moneyed aristocracy, are fitted up in very elegant style. The expense of living in such hotels is high, the system of boarding being in general not customary on the continent. The proprietors charge a certain price for rooms and meals, adding various sums for a great many little extras, in the shape of candles, service, &c. Hotels frequented by English travellers are the most comfortable ; they have reading-rooms, good clean beds, and comfortable arrangements. Their charges are somewhat higher than those of the other hotels, but travellers who do not hesitate to spend a little more money for the sake of cleanliness and comfort, should stop at these. However, there are everywhere good hotels, patronized by the better classes of society, where moderate prices are charged, and where guests receive more attention than at the so-called first class hotels. The rule for patients is, to remain at the hotel no longer than necessary to find furnished apartments, of which plenty can be had at every watering place; the inhabitants, in order to gain as much money as possible, give up their best rooms to the visitors, while they themselves take up their abode in small garret-rooms. The prices of rooms vary according to locality, outfit, and season. Elegant rooms can be had in handsome villas, for which a handsome price is charged; but there are many others, fully answering all reasonable demands, which are let at moderate prices. In fact you can live just as you choose. Even in the most fashionable spas, as for instance, Baden-Baden, Homburg, &c., you can live economically.

Highly interesting to every visitor of the larger watering places is the great variety of the society which assembles there. Places like Wiesbaden, Karlsbad, Baden-Baden, can really be styled *world baths*. There, in the height of the season, you find representatives of all nations of the globe; promenading in the *Kurgarten* or under the colonnades, you hear conversation carried on in all the languages of the civilized world. Distinction of rank and class seems to have disappeared for a short time; persons who at home would hardly recognize each other, here meet on neutral ground in a friendly and genteel manner. Proud kings and potentates walk unceremoniously among humble plebeians, great statesmen, profound scholars, celebrated artists, rich nabobs, poor school-teachers, broad shouldered peasants, and last, but not least, celebrities of the *demi-monde*, all mixed promiscuously, united by the common desire to amuse themselves as well as possible during the time of their involuntary sojourn. I say involuntary, because the majority of visitors, particularly those who are truly ailing and undergo a strict treatment, rejoice when the day of departure arrives, and with it, as they often foolishly believe, the liberty to again indulge in former irregularities of living. There is another class of bath visitors, whom one might rather call *fancy patients;* they flock to the watering places, only because it is the fashion to do so. Belonging to the wealthier classes of society, they particularly patronize the elegant, fashionable Rhenish spas, where they are sure to meet the best and most select company, the *élite* of the European society. Gay and joyful fugitives from home, they drink a few glasses of mineral water in the morning, merely as a matter of form, and devote the remainder of the day to pleasure and amusement. The Bohemian spas—Karlsbad, Marienbad, &c.—although not less frequented, have the reputation of being chiefly visited by such patients as are really in need of careful medical treatment, and who generally pass through a regular and often even severe, bath course.

No complaint can reasonably be made of the public morality at the German watering places, since the gambling-houses have been closed. Decency and good manners prevail everywhere ; only those can find fault who disapprove of all kinds of amusements, however innocent, and who always grumble and growl at the immorality of our time, while in reality for hundreds of years society has not reached such a high standard of morality as it nowadays enjoys. It was not so in the good old times. The celebrated Poggio has given an amusing description of bath life in the fifteenth century. At that time the baths undoubtedly were the seat of great immorality and licentiousness ; men and women, boys and girls, were in the habit of bathing together, perfectly nude, and behaved in the most disgraceful manner. The practice of ladies and gentlemen bathing together in large swimming-baths still prevails in some places ; as in Leuk (Switzerland), Baden (near Vienna), Neuhaus and Tüffer (Styria), &c.; but each bather must wear a long bathing-gown, and not the slightest indecency ever occurs.

As a general feature of the various baths the *bazaars* deserve to be mentioned, for which, in some places—as Wiesbaden, Beichenhall, &c.—very handsome buildings have been erected. They are an accommodation for the visitors, and an inducement to spend their money for a good many handsome, and sometimes useful, but at all events not very cheap, articles—be they those pretty knick-knacks, or notions, exhibited equally as good and cheap in the brilliant show-windows of the Strand or Oxford Street, or on Broadway ; or fancy articles manufactured as a specialty at the particular place; or like the Sprudel stones at Karlsbad, or those elegantly framed oil-pictures, offered at many spas as genuine Canalettos or Tintorettos, but in reality inferior copies, of no value.

This is the general appearance of a continental spa. To keep the various institutions in good order, to make new improvements, to engage well-trained bands of music, requires a considerable outlay of money. In order to defray these expenses, every person residing above a week at a watering place, must pay a small fee, called *Kurtaxe*, for which sum he obtains the right of free entrance to the conversation-house, reading-rooms, &c., and the privilege of drinking as much of the mineral waters as he pleases. Different prices are charged for the baths; tickets are sold for first, second, and even third class baths, the first class being a little more elegant: a considerable reduction is usually made to those who buy a dozen tickets. At some places, as for instance at Karlsbad, higher charges are stipulated for baths taken from seven a.m. to three p.m., than for those taken later. At most of the spas the bathing-rooms, especially of the first class, are handsomely fitted up, the tubs being constructed of marble or porcelain; well-trained and courteous waiters are everywhere in attendance. Baths taken in large basins in company with others are cheaper than single baths, but not to be recommended, as the bathers are wrapped in long bathing-gowns which prevent the water from coming in close contact with the skin, whereby it loses much of its efficacy. A popular prejudice exists in regard to common baths, based on the belief that one may there contract some contagious disease : this seems to be erroneous, as we have no proof that such has ever occurred.

CHAPTER V.

BATH LIFE AND BATH RULES.

BE regular in all your doings; rise early, retire early, eat and drink moderately, and, if possible, always at the same hour of the day; be constantly in the open air, and do not trouble your mind with business affairs. These are the principal rules of bath life.

From six to eight in the morning the patients gather around the fountains, each one armed with a porcelain cup, or a glass, holding from six to eight ounces of water. The fountains are generally covered by structures in the shape of small pavilions or temples. In some spas, as, for instance, in Homburg, they are uncovered and surrounded by splendid marble work. Long colonnades, either of marble or iron, are annexed, protecting patients, while drinking, from rain or sunshine. Here they stand in long rows, one behind the other, waiting patiently for their turn, ladies and gentlemen promiscuously, no preference being given either to the fair sex, or to the aristocrat, or to the proud priest; all are alike before the goddess of the fountain, represented by a young girl, who will speedily fill your cup, as soon as you have a chance to approach her. Then you step aside and slowly drink the water, while either standing or sitting, but not walking or chatting. Some persons, fearing the water may injure the teeth, prefer to sip it through a glass tube. This is hardly necessary, as no mineral water contains substances strong enough to corrode the teeth ; but if the water is very hot there is no harm in observing this precaution.

If you go early to the well you have the advantage of being served promptly, otherwise you are often obliged to stand in a line with several hundred persons, advancing slowly, until at last the fountain is reached ; and that annoyance must be endured four, five times, and oftener, according to the number of cupsful you have to drink. The time-honoured practice of drinking early in the morning is no fancy, but has a rational basis. Because, not only is the cool, bracing morning air highly beneficial to the patients, especially to those who drink hot springs, but, what is most important, the stomach then is empty, and best prepared to digest and absorb the mineral water. Full-blooded persons, and those inclined to perspire freely, should always go early to the fountain, especially if they drink hot waters. The rule not to take any nourishment before going to the well should not be too strictly applied to weak invalids, who may take a cup of coffee or tea as a stimulant, in order to strengthen themselves for their morning task. It is customary to drink the water at intervals of fifteen, twenty, or thirty minutes, in order to give the stomach sufficient time to digest it. To promote the absorption, patients promenade under the colonnades, or in the *Kurgarten ;* but they should not walk fast, nor should they overheat themselves, as so many over-zealous persons are in the habit of doing. After the usual interval of fifteen minutes another cup of the water may be taken; but if a sensation of fulness in the stomach is felt, it is better to wait ten or fifteen minutes longer. Sometimes cold mineral waters are not well tolerated by the stomach; in this case they should be warmed, for which purpose the necessary appliances are everywhere provided. To increase the medicinal effect of the waters, many patients, particularly those affected with bronchial diseases, mix them with warm milk or whey. The number of glasses to be taken must be determined by the bath doctor; it varies according to the nature of the disease, the age and constitution of the patient, and the absorbing power of the stomach. There are many patients who, erroneously believing that the larger the quantity of water they drink the quicker must be the recovery, flood the stomach with immense quantities. But they are greatly mistaken. *Nature will never submit to our arbitrary dictates.* A feeble condition usually takes hold of the patient who drinks excessively; nausea, dyspepsia, loss of appetite, are symptoms of the deranged digestion. The nutrition is impaired, congestion of the brain, and even apoplexy, often occur. As soon as the first of these symptoms is noticed the patient must stop drinking for a few days, and then recommence with a very small quantity.

Having finished your morning task by swallowing the prescribed quantity of water, you must take a walk of about an hour before taking breakfast. This exercise is necessary, as a stomach expanded by water is not able to digest food. By promenading you promote the absorption of the mineral water, and increase your appetite. But *promenading* does not mean *running*. Many patients spoil their health by running about in the woods every morning, returning to the breakfast-table exhausted and overheated. Coffee or tea, with one or two rolls, and one or two soft-boiled eggs, are quite sufficient for breakfast. Fish, meat, or hot cakes should not be taken. The English, being very exclusive, generally take breakfast at their hotels or lodging-houses. Far more preferable is the German custom of resorting to a garden restaurant. To sit there sipping the delicious high-flavoured coffee, nowhere else so well prepared as at the large watering places of Central Europe, while inhaling the fresh, bracing morning air, among hundreds of other visitors, every one coming provided with a paper-bag filled with fresh Vienna rolls, is indeed one of the charms of German bath-life. The Austrian spas are especially celebrated for having the best coffee gardens, an unsurpassed coffee, and excellent Vienna bread—so excellent, indeed, that many patients cannot withstand the temptation of eating too much of it, thereby frequently producing indigestion. And here it also seems appropriate to admonish against eating those rich and quite indigestible cakes (*Pretzels*) offered for sale by the bakers at most of the watering places.

The morning and evening hours being generally very cool on the continent, patients should dress accordingly. They should always wear *flannel undershirts*, even on very warm days, as the weather often suddenly changes from warm to cold. For the same reason they should always be provided with a shawl or an overcoat. Being mostly out-doors, promenading in the woods or shady walks, they feel inclined to sit down from time to time to enjoy a short rest, or to stop on some elevated point to take a view of the surrounding scenery. The perspiration being always increased by the exercise, they are very apt to take cold, if not prepared to make immediate use of a wrap. This happens so frequently, particularly during the warm summer days, that every bath doctor should direct the special attention of his patients to this subject. It is surprising how careless the latter are in this respect. To carry a shawl is too troublesome; but they forget that a catarrh caused by suppressed perspiration is far more troublesome, and sometimes even dangerous. Ladies while drinking the mineral water should not wear their corsets or dresses too tight, as this would prevent the stomach from expanding, especially if the water is rich in carbonic acid.

After breakfast it is expedient to walk a short time, and to rest thereafter until noon. Dinner is usually taken at one o'clock. In many watering places, especially in Germany and Switzerland, the fashion of *table d'hôte dinners* prevails, in my opinion a very undesirable practice. As a general thing, patients eat too much at these dinners—the variety of dishes, and the length of time spent at the table, enticing them to fill their stomachs with a load of indigestible food. This especially refers to a certain class of patients, who at home live on a small scale and on a scanty diet; these, delighted by the novelty of sitting at a large, opulent table, in the company of fashionable society, are too much inclined to yield to the temptation, and to indulge too freely in the consumption of ragouts, heavy puddings, and all kinds of compound dishes which compose the unwholesome fare at a first class table d'hôte. Ladies should keep in mind that they considerably impair the digestion by going to the table d'hôte *en grande tenue*. In full dress, the stomach is so compressed by corsets and dresses, that its functions can hardly be performed. These so very popular table d'hôte dinners should be abolished, they being inimical to health, and one of the principal causes of indigestion. To be sure, many patients participate in them merely for the purpose of taking their repast in company with the well educated, refined class of people who usually assemble at these table d'hôtes. But they can meet with such society just as well at the large restaurants where dinners *à la carte* are served. In the Austrian watering places table d'hôte dinners are not customary, to the great advantage of the patients; nor are dishes unfit for patients under treatment by mineral waters allowed to be put on the bill of fare. Almost all patients eat *à la carte*, and order such dishes as agree with their constitution and the nature of their disease. On the whole, according to my experience, the cooking in Austria is plainer and more wholesome for invalids than that in Germany, where too much fat, or butter of a dubious quality, is used in preparing the victuals.

After dinner a moderate exercise is again recommended. Old or weak persons may rest a short time; a little nap on an easy chair, or on a bench under a shady tree, is not so dangerous as still believed by many bath doctors, who indeed consider any sleep after dinner a fearful violation of that old bath rule which strictly forbids such a *siesta* as extremely hazardous. There is no doubt that to full-blooded persons, with an apoplectic habit, a long sleep after dinner may prove injurious, as during that time the digestion is in full action, and congestion of the brain easily occurs; but such persons should at all times abstain from sleeping after a heavy meal, especially on warm, close days, on which the propensity to cerebral congestion is increased.

There are many patients who, having hardly finished their dinner, hasten away to run about in the woods, or to climb as many hills as possible, erroneously believing thereby to facilitate the digestion. Especially those who pass through a bath course for the first time, are mostly under the impression that a great deal of exercise, combined with profuse perspiration, is absolutely necessary for the success of the treatment; they very often overdo the work by zealously running about the whole afternoon until late in the evening, climbing up and down the surrounding hills and mountains until fatigue and exhaustion force them to return to their residence. Such excessive exercise is injurious, and should never be indulged in, not even by strong persons. All extreme habits are unfavourable to the success of the treatment; to keep the "golden mean" is an old rule, which should be adhered to by patients even more strictly than by others. We therefore repeat, as the principal rule of bath life, proclaimed with singular unanimity by all bath physicians, take constant but moderate exercise in the open air, alternating with intervals of rest and recreation. Patients should stroll on the shady promenades of the *Kurgarten*, walk through the forests, especially through pine woods, and may also climb hills of moderate elevation, the latter exercise being even more profitable than promenading on the plain, as it requires a little more exertion, and accelerates the circulation of the blood and the peristaltic action of the bowels. Moreover, the view of a pleasant scenery, varying as often as another high point is reached, is animating and exhilarating to the mind of the patients, who soon become wearied by the monotony of bath life. " Bodily exercise," says Braun, " strains on all branches of the organic life—as the consumption and reproduction of muscular tissue, which is manifested by the growing muscular power, and the increase of the urea, and the chloride of sodium of the urine ; the promotion of the respiratory process, which is permanently increased by the growing power of the respiratory muscles ; the activity of the function of the skin and all glandular organs ; the augmentation of hunger and of the supply of food, and consequently of the digestion and assimilation of the nutriments— the result of all this being a better nutrition of the blood and the tissues."

Excursions on a small scale are very recommendable ; the bodily exercise connected with them, the change of air and scenery, always exert a beneficial influence on the body and the mind of the patient.

But such little trips should not be converted into extended railway excursions, from which the patient returns so fatigued and exhausted that he is hardly able the next morning to rise and to walk to the spring. Such a practice, though very often indulged in, is imprudent.

The principal and most agreeable entertainments for most of the patients, and the best way to spend part of the afternoon, are the regular concerts given by the band (*Kurkapelle*) of the spa in the public parks. This is the time and place for the general reunion of the visitors, who go there to see and to be seen, and to take their afternoon coffee. A great many patients are in the habit of again overloading the stomach with a large number of cakes or rolls; they should not eat any such things so soon after dinner. There is no objection to taking coffee in the afternoon, as it may somewhat assist the digestion if taken without, or at least with very little, cream; but to eat pastry again is a noxious practice on the part of invalids, whose digestive power is impaired by the daily draughts of large quantities of mineral water.

After the concert, patients may again take a little walk, and after taking a light supper should retire early, in order to have sufficient time for a sound, long sleep, which is the best means of refreshing and invigorating themselves.

All mental labour and excitement must be strictly avoided, the mind needing rest just as well as the body. Therefore, when you leave your house, give orders not to trouble you with business affairs. To read a long time in a close and ill-ventilated reading-room is not advisable. If you cannot do without reading, take your newspaper, or some other light reading matter, and glance over it while sitting on a pleasant resting-place in the woods or gardens, always keeping in mind that fresh air is the elixir of life. Extensive letter-writing is decidedly pernicious ; by sitting at the desk and writing you compress the stomach and intestines, and impede the digestion. I especially call the attention of the ladies to this point, as many of them are in the habit of attending to their correspondence late in the evening, and of spending several hours in writing long letters. A restless night, a sleep disturbed by vague dreams, head-ache, and general relaxation, are the results of the excitement produced by such a practice.

I cannot refrain from denouncing another bad practice, very much indulged in at some of the large watering places, as Karlsbad, Marienbad, Kissingen, &c., viz., that of playing cards or chess for several hours after dinner. The excitement of the game, and the loss of proper exercise after the principal meal of the day, combined with a lengthy stay in an ill-ventilated, warm room, which generally is filled with smoke and impure air, must necessarily exert a detrimental effect on the digestion.

It remains to say a few words on the theatre and the dance. While of themselves an occasional dance, or attendance on theatrical performances, might not be injurious, still I consider both entertainments unsuitable for invalids. A crowded theatre, filled with a vitiated, foul air, is not a suitable place for sick persons, who, by leaving it in a state of high perspiration, as it is usually the case, expose themselves to the danger of catching a severe cold. The same can be said of the dancing. To remain several hours in an over-heated dancing-room, whose air is impregnated with dust, and with the exhalations of a large crowd of dancers, is not beneficial to patients, be they anæmic young girls who are longing for some better blood and red cheeks, or asthmatic gentlemen greedy of an abundance of fresh air, or hysterical ladies with a deranged nervous system. It is fresh, pure air, which they all constantly need, day and night; while all crowded, ill-ventilated, and over-heated rooms are noxious and insalubrious.

Finally, I should like to speak of the company patients should select during their sojourn at the spa, a subject really not so unimportant as many are apt to think. Pleasant and cheerful company has a great influence on the mind of the patient, it makes him feel livelier and happier; and it is a fact, that animated and hopeful persons have a greater chance of recovery than those of a hypochondriacal disposition and a depressed mind. Single persons often feel lonesome and uneasy among the crowd of strangers they find at the large spas; especially do Englishmen and Americans who are unacquainted with the German language, find it very difficult to pick out some suitable companions. Those who speak German have a wider range of selecting proper company, and will easily find some congenial persons with whom they can harmonize during the short time of their sojourn. Do not associate with patients who entertain you with long stories of their own complaints, or of similar ailments of their relatives up to the tenth or fifteenth generation ; nor with those who give you detailed accounts of innumerable cases exactly like yours, which have not been cured at the spa, and had ended fatally. Such melancholy company is of no advantage to you. Try to find one of those merry, jovial, well educated persons who are in the habit of frequenting all the large watering places by the hundred, always prepared and eager for a spirited, interesting conversation which will animate and enliven you. Avoid speaking of business and its troubles, and turn all your attention exclusively to one point, viz., to find out the best way of spending time and money in a pleasant and cheerful manner—as a merry, contented mind contributes a great deal to the success of the treatment.

At some baths the drinking is the principal object of the treatment, at others it is the bathing ; if both are practised, the bath is usually postponed until after breakfast.

In order to get a bath at a convenient time, every patient should give notice early in the morning on the day he wishes to bathe, or rather the day before, taking care that his name be booked at the office of the bath direction, otherwise he may not get a bath until late in the afternoon, or even one at all. Places of great reputation, as Karlsbad, Teplitz, Gastein, &c., are so crowded in the height of the season, that patients must make arrangements for their baths several days in advance. There are many patients who prefer to bathe early in the morning, when the stomach is empty. This rule may be a good one for strong persons; but old and debilitated persons, or those already fatigued by their morning task of drinking and promenading, should not bathe without having taken a light breakfast; attacks of vertigo, nausea, or fainting, often seize those who neglect this precaution. At all events, the best time for taking a bath is about an hour after breakfast, the hours from 9 to 12 A.M. being the most convenient. Those who are obliged to bathe in the afternoon should wait at least fully three hours after dinner. If possible, they should bathe regularly at the same hour every day, and all mental and bodily excitement must be carefully avoided. Therefore, extensive walks should not be undertaken before the bath; they are fatiguing, and might induce you, when the time for bathing approaches, to hurry, and thereby excite yourself. Nothing is more dangerous than to go into a warm bath with a quickened pulse and an over-heated circulation of the blood, which easily results in congestion of the brain, and even apoplexy.

The temperature of the bath must be determined by the bath physician; it varies according to the nature of the disease and the constitution of the patient. Anæmic and old persons can endure a higher temperature than plethoric and young ones. Those afflicted with lung or heart diseases should not take hot baths. The bath attendants being often not very particular about the temperature when preparing the bath, it is always expedient to examine it by the thermometer, and if not correct, to secure the proper temperature by admitting the necessary quantity of hot or cold water.

The duration of the bath must likewise be determined by the bath physician ; the chemical composition of the water, the age and constitution of the patient, and the nature of the disease, are the points to be taken into consideration. In the beginning of a bath course, twenty or twenty-five minutes are considered a sufficient time for a bath, afterwards thirty or forty-five minutes are allowed, but very rarely is the time extended to one hour. The only place on the continent where baths of longer duration are taken is Leuk, in Switzerland, where the patients remain several hours in the common baths, conversing, chatting, playing cards, &c. Ladies and gentlemen bathe here together ; but, as I have already remarked in a former chapter, such a practice is not desirable, as the bathers are obliged to wear long bathing-gowns, which prevent the mineral waters from coming in close contact with the skin. Single baths are, therefore, preferable ; or where large common swimming baths exist, they should be made more efficient by having separate hours for ladies and gentlemen respectively, in which case the long bathing dresses could be replaced by some other and more simple costume.

After the bath the patient should rub himself until perfectly dry, dress quickly, and repair to the reception-room, to rest there for a short time. If the weather is warm and pleasant, a short walk may then be taken ; but if moist and damp, it is better to go home and rest a short while. Warm clothing is always to be cared for, the skin being very sensitive after the bath. Persons subject to congestions of the brain should keep a cold wet towel on their heads, as long as they remain in the bath; for these as well as for debilitated or nervous patients, it is advisable not to bathe without having an attendant at hand to assist them in case of need. Patients should also abstain from sleeping in the bath, the temptation therefore being greatly increased by the soothing influence of the warm water on the nerves. A profuse perspiration after the bath is often very advantageous to a certain class of patients, especially to those affected with rheumatism, gout, secondary syphilis, &c.: bathers can easily produce perspiration by going home soon after the bath and covering themselves with a heavy blanket, in which they should remain for one or two hours. Ladies should not take hot baths during pregnancy and certain periodical indispositions. Hæmorrhages of any kind always forbid the use of hot baths.

The *number* of baths to be taken depends on the effect which they produce on the disease, and the constitution of the patient, the bath doctor being the competent person to decide this important question. In some cases the beneficial effect is very soon and strikingly manifested; in others it is hardly noticed during the whole bath course. In all watering places the regular course consists of twenty-one baths. It is hard to tell what has led to such an arbitrary and irrational rule, as it is quite impossible for a physician, no matter what remedy he might apply, to tell the patient beforehand how long it will take before the desired effect can be obtained. Still this rule yet exists, and many bath doctors adhere to it. The majority of cases treated by them being chronic, and generally of long duration, it is evident that twenty-one baths will be insufficient to effect a cure. How can patients, suffering for many years from severe attacks of rheumatism, gout, nervous head-ache, &c., reasonably expect to be freed from their ailments by a course of twenty-one baths? An intelligent patient, not believing in this irrational dogma, therefore will not despair when he sees no favourable result after having taken that ominous number of baths, but will go on with the treatment, and persevere as long as his judicious medical friend shall advise him to do so, and his power of endurance will permit.

To take more than one bath a day is of no benefit; for weak persons one bath every other day is often quite sufficient. The bathing-rooms should be high, airy and well ventilated; and every bather on entering a room which has been used a short time before, should satisfy himself that fresh, pure air has been admitted. This is often neglected when the number of bathers is very large. When the weather is damp and cold, it is very agreeable to have the room heated, and the sheets and towels with which the patient is to rub himself, warmed by little copper or tin appliances, provided for at every watering place.

To postpone the bath on account of unfavourable weather is hardly necessary, every patient being able to protect himself against the inclemency of the tremperature by proper clothing, or by riding in a carriage to the bathing-house.

After a number of baths have been taken, a rash, called the *Badfriesel*, frequently appears on the skin, especially if the water is heavily impregnated with salt. Formerly this rash was considered a critical symptom, and the first sign of improvement, and was as such eagerly looked for both by patients and doctors. However, it is nothing else than an irritation of the skin, caused by the salts contained in the mineral water, and has no essential effect on the disease; but in order to avoid the increase of this unpleasant irritation, the baths must be omitted for a few days. A large number of patients leave the spas entirely cured without having experienced the slightest attack of the *Badfriesel*; while others, who had been extremely tormented by severe eruptions, do not notice any improvement of their maladies. "The time has passed," says Dr. Valentiner, "when patient and doctor rivalled in their delight over an eruption on the skin, after the use of the baths: that beautiful time of the illusory bath crisis is passed, since we have come to regard these eruptions as mostly very unwelcome consequences of an irritation produced by the baths."

Another affection often produced by drinking or bathing, is the so-called *Brunnenfieber* (well-fever); a heavy head, restless nights, chills alternating with heat and followed by perspiration, excited pulse, are the symptons. Moreover, patients begin to dislike the water, the appetite, often increased by the treatment, fails, and the evacuation of the bowels becomes irregular. The system is believed to be saturated by the water, and this saturation is considered the cause of this febrile affection, which rapidly passes away if the treatment is interrupted for a few days.

The duration of the treatment by mineral springs cannot be determined beforehand ; it depends on the nature of the disease, and the susceptibility of the patient for the action of the mineral water. Some drink and digest it very well, others soon become disgusted with it, and are obliged to stop drinking ; on some the waters re-act very rapidly and effectively, while others, during the whole time of the treatment, hardly experience any effect at all ; some very soon have the sensation of being saturated by the water, others can take it for months without noticing any uneasiness. These and other considerations will guide the bath doctor when consulted by the patient, who on his own responsibility should neither alter, nor shorten, nor prolong the cure.

It is the practice of many bath physicians when commencing the treatment to limit it beforehand to four weeks ; perhaps the experience that the *Brunnenfieber* (well-fever) often appears at this time has led to that practice, which nevertheless is wholly arbitrary. No physician can ever pretend to be able to define the time necessary for the cure of a chronic disease, without running the risk of being considered a humbug. The principal rule for the invalid is to be patient, and for the bath doctor not to yield to the impatience of his patient. I especially recommend to Americans, who are obliged to undertake such a long and expensive voyage in order to reach a European spa, not to break off the bath course too early; a few weeks more devoted to the goddess of the fountain will often prove of considerable benefit. It is generally known that hardly any disease of long standing can be permanently cured by a medication of four or five weeks; why should we expect that such a miracle can be performed by the drinking of a mineral water, however powerful it be? If a patient is tired, after having passed through a course of four weeks without having yet obtained the desired result, he may stop for a month or two, and then recommence another course. A good many patients are in the habit of doing this; and I should advise Americans who do not intend to visit Europe a second time, to follow the same method. I often had the opportunity, during my stay at Karlsbad and other spas, to impress upon the minds of visitors, especially Americans, the necessity of remaining long enough to give the spring a fair chance of showing its effectiveness; and I had the satisfaction of seeing them pleased with the result. I have also met quite a number of English and Americans who had been visiting the spas for several years in succession in order to become permanently cured, which is the proper way of doing, because, if you come to the conclusion that the first trial has done you good, and you have full confidence in the efficacy of the spa, I positively advise you to try it again. *No sacrifice is too great for the sake of health and happiness!*

CHAPTER VI.

THE DIET DURING THE BATH CURE.

A GREAT many stringent rules have been laid down in regard to the diet during the bath treatment, and a great deal of redtapeism has for a long time prevailed in those things. Undoubtedly a proper diet is of greater importance than most of the patients are aware of. Every intelligent physician knows that in the treatment of chronic diseases by dietetic advice he often obtains far better results than by large bottles of medicine. But how few of our patients are willing to submit to the rigid dietetic rules of the family physician! Nevertheless, strange as it may appear, as soon as they are away from home, and under the care of a bath doctor, they usually yield to his dictates, by giving up their favourite dishes and drinks. For every chronic disease a special diet must be ordained; and no intelligent patient will indulge in a large quantity of indigestible food so long as he is obliged to take medicine. We should, therefore, expect to see this rule strictly adhered to by those who, while undergoing a bath treatment, fill their stomach every morning with a considerable quantity of mineral water. But a great many have neither the common sense nor the energy to withstand the allurements of the stomach; and I believe this undeniable fact has contributed a great deal to establish so many rigid rules for patients at watering places, which we to-day consider irrational or immaterial. The old bath doctors were very well aware that the more the whole bath life was surrounded with a mysterious nimbus, the greater would be the influence they could exert on the minds of their patients, and the less would be the opposition made to their directions, even by those who at home would not at all follow the conscientious advice of their family physician. We should not too severely criticize our old colleagues for ostracizing many articles of food, perfectly harmless when taken in moderate quantity. They knew the human heart, and the carelessness of the patients in regard to diet, and therefore considered it safer and better for the success of the treatment, and the welfare of their *protéges*, to submit them for a short time to a rather despotic dietetic regimen. It is really astonishing how often the simplest dietetic rules are violated by injudicious patients. For instance, every person of common intelligence is well aware that no heavy meal should be taken shortly before going to bed; nevertheless, at all the watering places those restaurants which have the reputation of having a good table are filled until late in the evening with patients, who overload the stomach with all kinds of food. Even in Karlsbad, which has the most powerful mineral water in Europe, and where the dietetic rules are more rigidly observed than at any other watering place, hundreds of patients indulge in opulent suppers. We should, therefore, not blame those medical attendants who, profiting by the experience of many years' practice, are apparently a little severe in regard to the diet. A restricted, scanty food at all events will hardly ever do much harm, while injudicious eating and drinking cause incalculable injury to many patients during every season. From my own experience, I must rather confess that the bath physicians nowadays often seem to pay too little attention to the subject of diet, neglecting to give their patients the proper advice, and to impress upon their mind the necessity of submitting to a proper dietetic regimen.

Although it is very difficult to lay down general rules on bath diet, as every patient and every mineral spring require a different regimen, I shall nevertheless endeavour to do so, for the information of those who are desirous of receiving some general knowledge on this important matter. However, the bath doctor must give special directions in each individual case, according to the nature of the disease, the age and constitution of the patient ; and last, but not least, in conformity with the chemical constituents of the water. It is obvious that patients affected with disorders of the digestive organs—and this class embraces perhaps the majority of all those who visit watering places—must be subjected to a quite different, and generally far more rigid diet, than others who are exhausted by loss of blood, or debilitated by defective nutrition. For the latter, a nourishing, invigorating diet is indicated ; while corpulent persons, addicted to a luxurious life, should be enjoined to give up their opulent table for some time, and to live on frugal rations, in order to prevent any further accumulation of superfluous fat.

The general rule for all patients, without exception, is to adhere to a *simple, frugal, and easily digestible diet ;* every patient taking medicine should follow this rule, and so much more should those do so who are under the influence of mineral waters, all of which tax the digestive organs in a high degree. Patients should bear in mind that they do not derive any benefit *from the quantity of food they consume, but from the quantity they digest and assimilate.* Their meals should consist of a few well-prepared, palatable dishes ; all luxuries of a grand table in the shape of rich preserves, desserts, &c., being excluded, as injurious to the digestion, and incongruous with the mineral water. The early rising and constant exercise in the open air increase the appetite, and induce many patients to eat more than they are able to digest ; for this very reason they should abstain from *table d'hôte* dinners, as already explained in the preceding chapter. A strict regularity in the time of taking meals is also very essential, and beneficial for the digestion ; however, patients are only too often induced to break this rule by their frequent visits to coffee-houses and places of amusement when promenading or on excursions. But they can easily avoid all irregularities by judiciously disposing of the time employed for such visits. In order to be sure of not overloading the stomach, they would do well to stop eating before their appetite is fully appeased, without, however, going to the other extreme of starving, which many imprudent patients consider indispensable for the success of the cure. The intelligent reader, understanding the true meaning of these rules, will steer safely between the Scylla of intemperance and the Charybdis of abstinence.

For a long time certain articles of food—as butter, fat, salads, fruit, even coffee and tea—were interdicted as incompatible with the chemical constituents of the mineral waters. Our knowledge of their chemical action having been greatly increased, the medical verdict against the use of these articles has been considerably modified. Fruit was proscribed, because the organic acids contained therein were believed to decompose the carbonate of soda, which is the principal constituent of the alkaline waters; for the same reason the verdict against salads was given. At present, we very well know that those acids do not counteract the chemical action of these waters, and should not on that account object to the moderate use of fruit or salads; but experience has sufficiently demonstrated that these articles of food, when taken during a bath course, have proved injurious by producing colic, diarrhœa, vomiting, &c.; therefore the bath physicians are fully justified in their unanimous veto of fruit and salads.

Fat and butter were also supposed to counteract the chemical action of the alkaline waters, but this is not the case. Nevertheless, fatty articles of food must be avoided on account of their indigestibility. The fat of meat, fish, lobsters, ducks, geese, are hard to digest by a stomach weakened by large draughts of mineral water. Moreover, there are a great many patients who should abstain from all fat and butter, these articles being especially inimical to their recovery, as for instance those affected with enlargement of the liver, gall-stones, obesity, &c. To others, as scrofulous or anæmic persons, the moderate use of butter or fat is rather beneficial.

I shall now briefly review the various articles of food, suitable or not suitable to patients under bath treatment. They are allowed to eat beef, veal, lamb, venison, pigeon, chicken, trout, and herring; while pork, goose, duck, smoked beef, corned beef, raw ham, sausage, eel, salmon, carp, crabs, lobsters, and oysters are forbidden. Rich gravy, profusely poured over the meat or poultry, as usually served at the German restaurants, and mostly prepared with lard or butter of inferior quality, is injurious, and should be banished from the table of patients. Pies and rich puddings must also be crossed from the bill of fare; and last, but not least, even ice-cream is strictly forbidden! Carrots, asparagus, cauliflower, spinage, young green peas, are good for patients; while cabbage, turnips, beans, which produce flatulency, are on the proscription list. Rice, mashed potato, barley, sago, when taken in moderate quantity, will do no harm; almonds, nuts, raisins, the favourite dessert at *tables d'hôte*, are indigestible. All vegetables should be well prepared; but without much butter or fat.

All kinds of liqueurs are strictly forbidden; one or two glasses of a light French or Austrian wine may be taken with advantage. If there is no contra-indication on account of the nature of the disease or the constitution of the patient, a glass of good, light beer will often prove beneficial, especially to weak persons; but nervous, irritable persons should not take either wine or beer, and not even tea in the evening. The practice of drinking a large quantity of soda or seltzer water at the meals prevails at most of the watering places, though it is not commendable. All waters containing carbonic acid expand the stomach and easily impair the digestive power ; therefore at meals they should be taken only in moderate quantity, and mixed with wine.

Three meals a day are the rule during the bath course—breakfast, dinner, and supper ; weak persons are sometimes advised to eat oftener, but only a small quantity at a time. For breakfast—tea, coffee, cocoa, milk, or chocolate may be taken, with one or two rolls, and one or two soft-boiled eggs; a plate of soup, taken a little later, is often beneficial. For dinner—soup, meat, and some light vegetables, are quite sufficient ; those who are in the habit of taking a cup of coffee (without milk) directly after dinner, may do so. In the evening, a scanty supper should be taken, which can easily be digested before the next morning, thus leaving the stomach empty, and well prepared to receive the usual supply of mineral water. A plate of soup, or two soft-boiled eggs with a roll, or a small portion of meat, compose a good supper for an invalid.

There are many persons who cannot sleep without having taken a glass of wine or beer ; in such cases a deviation from the general rule forbidding those drinks in the evening, is allowed. "Even the most general and approved rules," says Braun, "permit individual exceptions, as for instance the verdict against late and copious suppers, as there are many patients, especially those suffering from nervous affections, who cannot sleep unless they go to bed while the process of digestion is going on, and others who cannot rest at all without having taken a sedative in the shape of a glass of wine or beer. Many physicians, always ready to give a dose of morphine to allay a restless patient, zealously object, because it is the custom to do so, to a glass of wine, though it is a more wholesome soporific."

Formerly patients who intended to go to a watering place were obliged to undergo a preparatory course of treatment. Purgatives, emetics, even venisections, were freely used, until the unfortunate victims were so much reduced in strength, and their digestion was so impaired, that after their arrival at the mineral spring they could not commence the bath course until the digestion had sufficiently improved by proper treatment. This practice has been abandoned by all intelligent practitioners, who simply advise their patients to be moderate in food and drink, and particularly not to gratify their greed for favourite dishes and drinks—a habit practised by many patients just before commencing the bath course.

A far greater importance is generally attributed by the bath physicians to the so-called *after cure*. It is evident, and every intelligent reader will coincide with me, that even the most successful treatment will be counteracted, and perhaps entirely frustrated, if the patient, after leaving the spa, soon relapses into his former irregular and often extravagant mode of living. What benefit can be drived from a cure of four or five weeks' duration, in however an energetic and efficacious manner it may have been carried on, if it is not followed up, and completed afterwards, by a corresponding hygienic regimen? I venture to aver, that the majority of patients, after having cheerfully submitted for several weeks to the rigorous rules of the bath diet, as soon as the last cup of mineral water is drunk and the treatment brought to the eagerly desired end, joyfully throw off all restraint. In order to make up for the lost time, they ardently relish the favourite dishes, puddings, fruits, &c., unmindful of the fact that the digestive organs, weakened by the use of powerful mineral waters, are not prepared to receive an unlimited supply of indigestible victuals. By such a practice they often spoil the beneficial effects of the bath course. These effects, some times not at all visible during the sojourn at the spa, often appear some weeks, and even months, afterwards. We can not presume these *after-effects* to be imaginary, as many dissatisfied patients, who have finished the regular bath course without seeing an immediate success, are very apt to believe. The experience of physicians and patients has demonstrated, that such after-effects really take place, if not counteracted by an unreasonable regimen after the termination of the treatment. To obtain the desired result, it is absolutely necessary for patients, after having left the spa, to keep up the usual bath diet for several weeks longer, and to return gradually to their accustomed food. And in order to effect a permanent cure, they should for a long time regulate their diet in a rational manner according to the nature of their disease. This is the true and effectual after-cure of an intelligent patient. I purposely urge this point, as I have seen so many patients, immediately after having finished a bath treatment, rush to the enjoyment of an Epicurean table.

Moreover, it is not expedient to return home from the spa too early, and to resume business, with all its cares and troubles, its labours and exertions. The system usually being relaxed, and even exhausted, and the mind to a certain degree in a state of excitement, after a protracted and energetic treatment, it is easily understood that a time of entire rest and recreation should precede the return to active life. It is therefore highly advantageous to sojourn for several weeks at a pleasant, healthful station, either on the seashore or in a mountain region. The numerous health resorts of Germany and Switzerland, mostly located on some elevated mountain range, afford plenty of opportunity to those who desire to spend a few weeks in a quiet, reasonable manner, enjoying all the comforts of life, fresh, pure air, and the company of that refined class of society which usually congregates at these places.

Many physicians advise their patients to undergo, as an aftercure, a second treatment at a chalybeate spring, or to repair to a sea bath, in order to invigorate and strengthen the system. But, wherever you intend to go, do not do so in haste; travel slowly, comfortably, by short stages, and do not make night trips, there being too much discomfort and exhaustion connected with them.

Many patients, desirous of spending their time in a useful manner, are in the habit of visiting, soon after a bath course, some of the principal cities of the continent, running through the art galleries from morning till evening, gazing at pictures and statues, or perambulating dusty streets in search of curiosities and antiquities; others hasten to the alpine regions, climb the highest peaks, and return home proud and elated over their great achievements, unaware that they have thereby almost annihilated the beneficial results of the bath course. The bath physicians unanimously condemn these practices, especially all exerting trips through mountain regions; while moderate exercise is just as earnestly recommended as during the bath treatment.

Patients who have taken a number of warm baths are very apt to take cold, the skin having become very sensitive for even the slightest change of temperature; they should therefore turn their special attention to their clothing, at all times wear warm flannel underclothing, and avoid all exposure, especially to the cool night air or the moist morning dew.

CHAPTER VII.

WATER AND AIR.

WATER and air are such important factors in our life, and have been and still will be so often mentioned in this treatise, that the reader may wish to gain a little more information on this subject. Let us therefore enter into a brief discussion on the physiological effects of common water and mineral water, used internally and externally, adding a few remarks on mountain and sea air.

1. *Internal use of Water.*

If you drink a large quantity of water which is not instantly absorbed, you feel oppressed as by a heavy weight. But absorption generally commences as soon as the water is taken, and if the stomach is empty, goes on very rapidly. The water is absorbed by the veins of the stomach and the intestines, but more by those of the former; the secretion of the saliva, bile, and urine, is increased. The maximum of the absorption is reached about two or three hours after the water has been drunk, the excretion by the kidneys being most abundant at that time. Water containing salts is not so rapidly absorbed as common water; the less salt it contains, the more easily it is absorbed. The quantity of water which the stomach is able to receive and absorb is immense; persons are reported to have swallowed 200, and even 300, ounces of mineral water every morning for several weeks. The quantity of water in the blood varies according to the amount of water drunk and absorbed. A large quantity produces an expansion of the blood-vessels, and an increase in the secretions of the skin, of the intestinal canal, and especially of the kidneys, which carry off the largest portion of the water. Much water-drinking diminishes the specific gravity of the urine, makes it thinner, and increases the quantity of the urine. The perspiration is also thereby increased, but this increase varies much, according to the temperature of the water and the air, and the active exercise of the person. Water, if properly administered, augments all the secretions of the system, and facilitates the change of tissue and the renovation of the body. Water of a high temperature is more easily absorbed and is more efficacious than water of the usual cool temperature. Too much water-drinking impedes the digestion, disturbs the secretions, and often produces dropsy.

Water taken in large quantity expands the stomach, the intestines, the blood-vessels, the biliary passages, and the bladder; it liquefies the contents of the intestinal canal, and thereby promotes the evacuation; it facilitates the circulation of the blood in the smaller vessels of the liver, lungs, and spleen, thereby preventing or relieving congestions of these organs. The expansion of the biliary passages and the bladder by water, greatly helps to facilitate the passage of gall-stones and gravel.

Water, by diluting the contents of the stomach and intestines, is of great benefit in the treatment of poisoning; by its solvent power it promotes the digestion, improves the assimilation, and increases the change of tissue. Some practitioners, believing that water by its solvent power could remove the lithic acid from the system and thus cure gout, were wont to order their patients to swallow enormous quantities; but the result being unsatisfactory, this treatment has been given up.

Cold water is a stimulant, and as such highly beneficial in the treatment of atony of the stomach and the intestines, and of defective digestion caused thereby; it also diminishes the irritability of these organs.

Warm water is used with great benefit in many painful affections of the stomach and the intestinal canal; it fluidizes its contents more thoroughly than cold water, augments the secretions, and promotes the absorption of morbid deposits.

If mineral waters are drunk, the larger portion of them is also absorbed by the stomach; especially are the gases which they contain rapidly carried into the blood, while the absorption of the mineral constituents is somewhat retarded. High temperature of the water, and active exercise, favour the absorption. Another portion of the mineral water passes through the alimentary canal, where it is partly absorbed, the rest being eliminated by the action of the bowels.

Mineral waters act as stimulants on the stomach, partly by their low temperature, partly by the carbonic acid contained in most of them ; by some of their mineral constituents, especially the carbonates of soda and magnesia, they also neutralize the acids of the stomach. Very important is the purgative action produced by waters containing sulphates of soda and magnesia, which stimulate the mucous membrane of the intestinal canal, thereby increasing the peristaltic action of the bowels. Other mineral waters, especially those containing carbonate of lime, have a tendency to produce constipation, and are useful in the treatment of chronic diarrhœa. Carbonic acid, the most important element of the majority of all mineral waters, is partly removed from the stomach by eructation, partly absorbed; its action on the nervous system is similar to that produced by the sparkling wine. Lightness of the head, followed by drowsiness. is the symptom, which disappears if the quantity of the carbonic acid is diminished by adding warm water or milk to the mineral water. Carbonated water, taken in moderate quantity, is refreshing, and acts as a pleasant stimulant on the stomach.

2. *External use of Water.*

Externally, water is mainly used in the form of baths. The effect of a bath depends on the temperature of the water. If the latter is high, say about 102° to 110°, the temperature of the body is increased about 3° ; if the temperature of the bath is as low as 66°, it reduces the temperature of the body about 2° within ten or fifteen minutes. A temperature of 88° to 95° is considered indifferent, as it does not change the temperature of the system, and can be indulged in for a considerable time without any harm.

The cold bath reduces the frequency of the pulse, produces contraction of the capillary vessels of the skin, which becomes cool and pale, and a flow of the blood to the internal organs, viz., to the brain, lungs, kidneys, &c. But as reaction takes place, after a short while the skin becomes red, and the pulse normal, or even more frequent than before. The symptoms produced by the rush of blood to the internal organs, resulting from the action of the cold water, are these : dizziness in the head, tremor of the limbs, oppression of the chest, and a small pulse.

Hot baths accelerate the circulation of the blood, produce a rush of blood to the surface of the skin, and an expansion of the whole quantity of blood contained in the blood-vessels ; thereby causing congestions and profuse perspiration. Diseases occasioned by suppressed perspiration and morbid organizations are benefited by these baths. The stimulative effect produced by the high temperature of the hot water often proves very beneficial in cases of paralysis. The high temperature is probably the sole efficacious element of the mud, peat, and sand baths which are so much patronized on the continent both by physicians and patients, although the heavy weight of these substances may also contribute a good deal to their beneficial action in some affections, as enlargement of the liver, thickening of joints, &c.

Indifferent baths, which have a temperature of 88° to 95°, do not have any material physiological effect on the circulation of the blood, or on the nervous system. But the experience of many years has proved them highly beneficial in cases of nervous irritability, neuralgia, sleeplessness, hysterical spasms, &c.

Very young persons, and old ones, not being strong enough to bring on a speedy reaction, should not take cold baths; nor should decrepid persons, or invalids affected with severe disorders of the digestive organs or with a high degree of nervous irritability, submit to a cold water treatment. Diseases of the heart, congestions and hæmorrhages of the lungs, apoplectic dispositions, are also contra-indications to the use of cold water.

Water charged with carbonic acid produces a very pleasant prickling or burning sensation on the surface of the skin, a flow of blood to the latter, and redness and fulness of the pulse; therefore, it seems that this gas, when used externally, acts as a stimulant on the skin. Some salts, as chloride of soda, chloride of lime, contained in many mineral waters, also produce a stimulating effect on the peripheral nerves. The stimulative action of the carbonic acid is quicker, but that of the salts lasts longer; these, after having penetrated the epidermis, seem to remain longer in the skin, and thereby to produce the stimulation of the nerves.

Alkaline waters have no more effect on the system than common water baths, their salts not being absorbed by the skin; they mollify the epidermis, thereby enabling us to remove impurities accumulated on the skin, and they prevent the pores from being obstructed by the secretions of the sebaceous and sweat glands.

The general effects of strong mineral water baths may thus be summed up: they increase the circulation of the blood in the skin, promote its nutrition, augment the secretions, and often produce eruptions on the skin.

A few words may be added on the important and highly interesting question, whether the mineral constituents of the mineral waters are absorbed by the skin or not. For a long time it had been taken for granted that they were absorbed; and patients, as well as physicians, were accustomed to attribute the beneficial effects of the baths to that absorption, an opinion which even nowadays prevails among the visitors of all the watering places on the globe; especially those who take iron baths are convinced that the invigorating effect experienced by their use is the result of the absorption of the iron by the capillary vessels of the skin. But this is not the case. At present, the best authors on balneology coincide *that absorption by the skin does not take place;* that the sebaceous secretion of the latter is an absolute obstacle to the absorption of any mineral constituent of the mineral waters; and that absorption can only be facilitated by removing the sebaceous secretion by means of scraping, soaping, high temperature, long duration, and frequent repetitions of baths.

There seems to be no doubt that all the benefit actually derived from the use of mineral water baths is a result of stimulation of the peripheral nerves, produced by their mineral constituents and their temperature, whereby the activity of the skin is increased, the nutrition of the system improved, the circulation of the blood accelerated, and the transformation and renewal of tissue materially promoted.

3. *Mountain and Sea Air.*

In ancient, as well as in modern times, the popular idea has always prevailed, that country air, and especially mountain and sea air, was purer and more salubrious than city air. Greeks and Romans repaired to their summer residences in the country and on the sea-shore as soon as the summer heat made them feel uncomfortable in their elegant city mansions. Their sea-baths were notorious for the elegance, extravagance, and licentiousness of the fashionable society. The temples of their gods, to which invalids often resorted in order to restore their health, were mostly situated in elevated, salubrious regions.

There is, indeed, a great difference between country and city air—a greater one than most people imagine. Our modern, over-crowded cities—filled with the smoke, coal-dust, and refuse of innumerable factories, warehouses, and slaughter-houses, the air impregnated with the impurities of gas-houses and oil-refineries, of dusty streets and dumping grounds—are rather hotbeds of all kinds of diseases than suitable domiciles for a sound and vigorous population. Sufficient circulation, of air, absolutely necessary for its purity and healthfulness, is impeded by the height of large warehouses, churches, tenement houses, and other edifices. It has been demonstrated by M. Pasteur, a celebrated French savant, and by other able scientists, that city air is impregnated with innumerable microscopical organisms, *germs*, which are the cause of the putrefaction and decay of organic substances, and probably of many, if not of all, contagious diseases. " It has been established beyond all doubt," says one of these scientists, "that these organic substances, be they gaseous products of putrefactive processes in the animal or vegetable kingdom, or vegetable germs, or microscopical animalcules floating in the atmosphere, do reach the lungs in the current of air inspired, and are there capable of doing great mischief." We may reasonably infer that city air, in consequence of the large congregation of people, and of the immense amount of all kinds of organic substances accumulated in houses and streets, and of other deposits subject to easy decomposition, should be more infected with these atmospheric germs than country air, which is supposed to be comparatively free from them. The air of the large glacier in Switzerland called *Mer-de-glace*, was found entirely free from germs; and this may be the case on all elevated points of 3000 feet and more.

Country air contains a larger quantity of ozone. Ozone is modified oxygen; it destroys foul gases emanating from decomposed organic matter. The more ozone the air contains, the purer and fresher it is. It is the purity of the country air which produces such a beneficial, vitalizing effect on invalids; the feeling of delight and refreshment which they enjoy when inhaling the fresh, pure, bracing mountain air is intense, especially if they have been for any length of time confined to a close, ill-ventilated room.

Mountain air is cooler than the air of the plains;

it is also thinner, the atmospheric pressure being diminished, and containing less oxygen. Therefore, when we take active exercise in the mountains our inspirations must naturally become deeper and more frequent, in order to inhale the necessary quantity of oxygen. The capacity of the lungs and the activity of the whole system being thereby increased, the assimilation and nutrition are improved.

The changes of temperature are more sudden in the mountains, the currents of air are stronger and change more frequently than in the plains. The higher the elevation, the cooler and fresher, and the more bracing and invigorating, is the air; and in the same proportion the evaporation of the body is increased. Active exercise in the mountains accelerates the action of the heart and lungs, increases the circulation of the blood and the perspiration, and improves the digestion and the change of tissue.

Very striking is the effect of the Alpine climate on the deranged digestion. Its beneficial influence is soon experienced in the action of the stomach; the appetite being already restored during the first days of residence in an elevated region, the stomach requires more food, and substances which formerly were not at all tolerated are quickly and thoroughly digested. By degrees the action of the intestines becomes more regular, diarrhœa and other disorders disappear, and obstructions of the liver, spleen, &c., are much relieved. Most apparent is the beneficial effect of mountain air in cases of nervous debility and irritability, and nervous prostration caused by overstrenuous mental labour. Persons broken down by business troubles, or by professional strain on their mental capacities, wonderfully recuperate even after a brief stay in an alpine region; appetite, sleep, and good-humour soon return, the muscular power increases, the abnormal nervous irritability disappears, and a sound, healthy exterior takes the place of the former sickly and decrepid appearance. The same beneficial influence is experienced by invalids who have been debilitated by malaria, wounds, or chronic diseases of any kind.

Sea air is free from the dust and other impurities of land air, and contains a greater quantity of ozone. Its temperature is more equable—in summer generally lower, in winter somewhat higher than that of the interior. The atmospheric pressure and evaporation are also greater. Sea air contains a large amount of saline particles. It acts highly beneficially on the process of blood-making and on the nutrition, improves the digestion, and invigorates the nervous system. Bronchial catarrhs are much benefited by the inhalation of the sea air, while in tubercular affections of the lungs many medical authors consider sea air injurious. Asthmatic patients often derive great benefit from a protracted sojourn on the seashore; sea air is also recommended in cases of anæmia, general atrophy, spinal irritations, neuralgia, rheumatism, and gout (Braun). Organic diseases of the stomach and the alimentary canal are not generally benefited by the use of sea air.

PART II.

TOPOGRAPHICAL REVIEW OF THE WATERING PLACES.

Introductory Remarks.

IN the second part of this guide I intend to give a topographical description of the *principal watering places* of *Germany, Austria, and Switzerland*. The number of spas in these countries being really enormous, I shall mention only those which are of *special interest to English and Americans*, either by their superior chemical qualities and curative effects, or by their great reputation and easy access. Places too remote to be easily reached, or without any special attraction, shall be omitted ; nor shall I describe the mineral springs of places like Friedrichshull, Püllna, &c., which cannot be styled *spas*, as their waters, though very powerful, are not drunk at the wells, but only exported.

Every day, I might say, a new spring is discovered in some part of Central Europe ; its virtues are praised and extolled in newspapers and periodicals, as a panacea for all evils ; its comfortable arrangements and low prices are conspicuously advertised, and its situation is described as a *non plus ultra* of beautiful scenery, purity of air, &c., &c.

We shall confine ourselves to the description of those places which, by the experience of many years, have had their reputation established in regard to efficacy and superior arrangements. A little more space shall be devoted to grand spas, like Karlsbad, Baden-Baden, Kissingen, &c., they being unique, either by the efficacy of their waters, or by their excellent situation, or by the superiority of their arrangements and other attractions. Commencing with those in the north-westernly part of Germany, we shall proceed to the others near the Rhine and in Middle Germany, concluding with those in South Germany; the wells in the eastern part, viz. in Silesia, shall be briefly noticed. A similar course shall be pursued with the Austrian and Swiss baths.

At each place the names of physicians and hotels, taken from the latest editions of travelling guides, especially Baedeker's, and medical almanacks, shall be given. However, I feel myself in duty bound to remark, that this shall not be looked upon as a recommendation of any of them ; *it is intended to be nothing more or less than a guide to aid those who arrive at a watering place as perfect strangers and totally unacquainted with the locality.*

English and Americans should not believe that only the large, celebrated and fashionable watering places, frequented by vast numbers of their countrymen, are the most preferable in regard to entertainment and social intercourse. This is not always the case; there are even in the remotest portions of the Styrian and Swiss alps a great many charming little spas, where they can spend their time very pleasantly, with less expense and perhaps with more benefit to their health. This wholly depends on the individual disposition of the patient.

A topographical description of spas, in the manner in which I propose to give it, has to my knowledge, never before been attempted by any writer; but though it may be a little monotonous, I rather believe that precisely in this manner the reader will soon and easily obtain a general knowledge of the position and arrangements of the principal spas.

Their chemical composition and therapeutic action shall be discussed in the third part of this treatise.

CHAPTER I.

THE WATERING PLACES OF GERMANY.

A GLANCE at the map of the watering places will show the principal German spas arranged in four groups.

The *first* of these comprises a small number situated in the north-westernly part of Germany, between the cities of Hanover, Paderborn, and Münster. To this class I number Nenndorf, Eilsen, Rehme (Oeynhausen), Pyrmont, Meinberg, Lippspringe, Inselbad, Driburg.

The *second* group, the largest of the four, embraces the bulk of the German spas, situated in the western and middle portion of Germany, near the banks of the Rhein and Main. The principal baths of this class are *Aachen* (Aix-la-Chapelle), Burtscheid, Neuenahr, Bertrich, *Kreuznach*, Ems, *Schwalbach*, Schlangenbad, *Wiesbaden*, Weilbach, Soden, *Homburg*, Nauheim, Wildungen, *Kissingen*, Bocklet, Brückenau ; most of these belonging to the most favoured and celebrated spas of Europe.

The *third* group is situated in Baden, Würtemberg, and Bavaria. At the head of this class ranks *Baden-Baden ;* Wildbad, Cannstadt, Kreuth, Reichenhall, belong to the same class.

The *fourth* group is exclusively composed of the Silesian baths in the eastern part of Germany; of these Salzbrunn, Warmbrunn, Landeck, Cudowa, Reinerz, deserve to be noticed.

Supposing our reader to have arrived at Bremen or Hamburg, we shall commence our trip from here to the first group of the German spas. Passing through Hanover, we reach by railway the little, but well reputed, spa,

NENNDORF, a small village with 800 inhabitants; it has powerful sulphur-springs; besides these, there are salt-baths in Nenndorf, the salt-springs of the neighbouring village *Sooldorf* being carried thither by subterranean pipes, and used for bathing. It is situated in a woody region, 220 feet above the sea, with a climate which though variable is temperate and healthy, and with a mean summer temperature of 64° F. The air is rather moist. The arrangements for bathing and inhalation are good. Number of visitors about 1200 annually.

Hotels: Stadt Hannover, Hotel Kassel.

Physicians: Dr. Erve, Dr. Neussel, Dr. Varenhorst, Grandidier.

Access: From London or Paris, *viâ* Cologne by the Cologne-Minden railway to Minden, Haste, Nenndorf.

Travelling westward by railway we reach, in about an hour, station Bückeburg, and thence, by an hour's stage-drive, the sulphur springs of

EILSEN. This is a small place with 400 inhabitants,

situated in an open valley 273 feet above the sea; with a mild and pure air, well sheltered from the north and east; owing to its efficacious mud baths it has become quite popular. Number of visitors: 2000.

Physicians: Dr. Möller, Dr. Wegener, Dr. Schönian.

From Bückeburg station we reach in seventy-five minutes

REHME-OEYNHAUSEN, a celebrated spa (a station of the Cologne and Minden railway). It is a little city in Westphalia with 2000 inhabitants, situated 166 feet above the sea, in a pretty valley, surrounded by high hills; the air is fresh, pure, and moderately moist, rich in ozone. About 3700 persons visit the spa during the season, and 60–70,000 baths are given. The heat there is not so oppressive in summer as at most of the other continental spas, the mean summer temperature being 66° F. Sudden changes of the latter are prevented by the surrounding hills. The arrangements for bathing are perfect in every respect. The bathing-house *for the thermal baths* is a grand building in modern style, very tastefully fitted up. We enter it by a large, domed rotunda, which reminds us of the celebrated Pantheon at Rome; close by is an elegant reception-room, where bathers take a short repose after the bath. The two wings on each side of the rotunda contain sixty-eight spacious bathing-rooms, provided with large, commodious wooden tubs; everything looks neat and clean. There is another bathing-house, with 35 bathing-rooms, called the *Soolbade-Haus*, where plain salt-baths are given, which contain no carbonic acid. The spa has a handsome *Kurhaus*, with a fine dining-*salon*, reading-room, &c.; a *réunion* takes place every Saturday. A large splendid park adjoins the *Kurhaus*, and many shady walks afford pleasant opportunity for active exercise, even on very warm days. A very interesting feature of the place is the large, domed inhalation-room, where patients inhale the atomized salt water. There is also a fountain where the mineral water is drunk, but as it tastes very salty, only a very small quantity can be taken. The place deserves to be more patronized by English and Americans.

Excursions can be made to the Siehl, Melbergen, the Kappenberg, Eidinghausen, Haus Gohfeld.

Hotels: Vogler's Hotel, Deutscher Kaiser, Victoria Hotel.

Physicians: Drs. Lehmann, Müller, Rinteln, Rohden, Sauerwald, Weihe.

Access: From London or Paris, *viâ* Cologne, on the Cologne-Minden railway directly to Rehme, or from Hamburg and Bremen *viâ* Hanover.

Starting from Hanover in a southernly direction we reach by a two-hours' ride the old and renowned iron spa,

PYRMONT, a little city with 1400 inhabitants, in the charming valley of the Emmer, 400 feet above the sea, surrounded by hills 1000 feet high. It is frequented by 12,000 persons annually; 45,000 iron baths and 27,000 salt baths are given. The principal promenade for the patients is a beautiful alley of linden-trees, 1000 feet long, the trees having already reached an age of 200 years; the *Kurhaus*, theatre, *cafés*, and numerous shops, are on this avenue. Nowhere else have I seen such a surprisingly fine park, with the most beautiful promenades of the oldest linden and chestnut-trees, as at Pyrmont. The little city presents a very fine appearance; a large number of handsome villas, surrounded by fine gardens, afford pleasant residences for the patients. The environs are charming. At the end of the large linden-alley the principal well, called *Hauptquelle*, breaks forth; it is covered by a handsome iron structure; close by is a covered walk, where patients promenade on rainy days. About fifty feet distant is the *Brodel*, covered by a glass cupola; the immense quantity of carbonic acid contained in this spring keeps the surface of the water in a continuous bubbling motion. The *Helenenquelle*, which is also very popular, is very pleasantly situated in the centre of the park; its water is very rich in carbonic acid, and has a pleasant taste. The bathing-house for the iron baths is a large, high, and airy building, with sixty-eight bathing-rooms; the tubs are excavations in the floor, lined with stone, slate, or marble. A small Russian vapour bath is also in the house. The other bathing-house, where the *Soolbäder* (saline baths) are given, is situated at the other end of the city, near the railway station; it contains forty-one bathing-rooms. Near by is the *Salzquelle* (salt spring), which is drunk, the water being very refreshing, and not very salty. A tramway carries patients from the city to the *Soolbad*. The

Kurhaus is an insignificant building with a large dining-*salon*, and a reading-room, where the London *Times* can be read. Peat and pine-needle baths are given at this spa. In the immediate neighbourhood is a cave filled with carbonic acid, similar to the celebrated cave near Naples.

Excursions are recommended: to the Sohelemberg, Königsberg, Friedensthal.

Hotels: Grosses Bade-Hotel, Stadt Bremen, Krone, Lippischer Hof.

Physicians: Drs. Seebohm, Lynker, Gieseken, Gruner, Köhler, Menke, Sorauer, Marcus, Wietz.

Access: From London and Paris, *viâ* Cologne and Paderborn directly to Pyrmont.

Half an hour distant from Pyrmont is the railway station Bergheim, and near it

MEINBERG, a village with 1500 inhabitants, in a pretty valley 650 feet above the sea, on the slope of the Teutoburg forest; it has a mild climate and good arrangements for bathing and drinking; its sulphur springs, and especially the sulphur mud baths, are highly recommended. There are several springs with a large quantity of carbonic acid, which is used for baths and inhalations. Number of visitors, about 800.

Hotels: Stern Rose, Sonne.

Physicians: Drs. Caspari, Niedreck.

Access: From Hanover by the Hanover-Altenbeck railway to Bergheim; from London and Paris, *viâ* Cologne and Paderborn to Bergheim, thence by stage.

From Bergheim we reach in fifteen minutes the old city of Paderborn, the oldest bishopric of Westphalia, founded by Charlemagne, and thence by stage to

LIPPSPRINGE, a spa which lately has come into great reputation for diseases of the lungs. It is a small town in Westphalia, with 2000 inhabitants, 375 feet above the sea, located in a sandy plain; protected against the north and north-east winds by the hills of the Teutoburg forest (1000 feet high); it has a mild, equable climate; the air is constantly moist on account of the numerous copious sources of the rivers Lippe and Jordan, which spring forth and take their course near the *Kurgarten*. The number of visitors is about 2000 annually. As usually, there is a *Kurgarten*, an *old* and a *new Kurhaus*, with a large number of furnished rooms for patients, and a bathing-house with twenty-three bathing-rooms. Special features of the place are a large *salon* of 5433 cubic feet, and several smaller ones of 1270 cubic feet, for the inhalation of nitrogen, the gases discharged from the mineral spring containing 87 per cent. nitrogen, the inhalation of which is considered very salubrious in lung diseases. The principal spring is the *Arminiusquelle*. Special attention is paid to diseases of the respiratory organs.

Excursions are not much favoured, as persons with diseased lungs should avoid fatigue and excitement.

Hotels: Altes und Neues Kurhaus, Hotel Wegener, Krieger, Concordia.

Physicians: Drs. v. Brunn, Bussen, Dammann, Frey, Holtz, Rohden, Sauer.

Access: From Hamburg or Bremen, by railway *viâ* Hanover to Paderborn ; from London or Paris, *viâ* Cologne to Paderborn, thence by stage.

By a pleasant walk of ten minutes from the old city of Paderborn we reach a large establishment, called

INSELBAD, which has several springs similar to those of Lippspringe. It is a sanitarium, patients receiving board and medical attendance at the establishment, which is under the able management of Brügelmann. There are two rooms for the inhalation of nitrogen, a bathing-house with twelve bathing-rooms, and a large swimming-bath. Mud baths are also applied. All arrangements are good and comfortable, and prices moderate.

From Paderborn by railway in forty-five minutes we reach

DRIBURG, an old celebrated iron spa, situated in a charming valley of the Teutoburg forest, 633 feet above the sea, surrounded by hills 1255 feet high ; the climate is mild and healthy, the air pure and invigorating. The arrangements for iron and sulphur mud baths are good. It is a good place for invalids fond of a quiet country-like resort.

This spa has two rival establishments : the *old bathing-house*, containing thirty-four bathing-rooms, and a large number of furnished rooms for the accommodation of patients, and the *new one*, called *Kaiser-Wilhelmsbad*, with ten bathing-rooms and twenty furnished rooms. Two of the iron springs, the *Haupt* and *Wiesenquelle*, belong to the former ; the

Kaiser-Wilhelm Stahlquelle, the richest in carbonic acid, belongs to the latter. The environs are very attractive.

Lodgings at the two bathing-houses, private houses, and at the hotels : Kothe, Fengerling, Englischer Hof.

Physicians : Drs. Brück, Hüller, Ricfenthal, Venn.

Access : From Bremen or Hamburg, *viâ* Hanover to Driburg; from London or Paris, *viâ* Cologne and Paderborn to Driburg, which is a station on the Altenburg-Halzminden railway.

We now commence our trip through the second group of the German spas.

AACHEN (Aix-la-Chapelle), the old imperial city of Charlemagne, is the first place which we visit. It is the most celebrated sulphur bath in Europe, situated in Rhenish-Prussia, near the Belgian frontier, 534 feet above the sea, in a pleasant valley. It has a mild and healthy climate. It is the oldest of all German watering places, the wells having been known and extensively used by the Romans. The number of inhabitants is 80,000. The attractions afforded by such a large city in the shape of theatres, concerts, antiquities, &c., combined with a mild climate, induce many patients to remain there and undertake a cure during the winter months, they having the advantage of living in the same buildings where they take the baths. The wells issue from the limestone in the centre of the city. About 20,000 persons are annually recorded on the list of visitors, and 100,000 baths are given during the season. There is a spacious *Kurhaus* with a magnificent new concert-hall, and a large reading-room (London *Times* and *Daily Telegraph*.)

The *Kurgarten* is small, but there are fine promenades all around the city, where invalids have plenty of opportunity for bodily exercise. In the morning patients drink the water of the *Elisabeth-Brunnen* in a large rotunda built in Doric style, and promenade in the small *Kurgarten* in the rear of the fountain, where the band plays every morning.

Aachen has eight bathing establishments with one hundred bathing-rooms, nine vapour baths, two *piscinæ* (swimming-baths) and inhalation-rooms. All the bathing-houses are the property of the city, and under the supervision of Dr. Lersch, the able author of a large number of excellent works on balneology. The most magnificent bathing-house is the *Kaiserbad*, one of the best arranged buildings of the kind in Germany, with perfect arrangements for bathing, and large *salons*, and elegantly furnished rooms for invalids. All the bathing-rooms are high and airy, the walls being tastefully covered with finely-coloured tiles. The bathing-tubs are excavations in the floor, built of bricks and cement, with marble steps and seats. There is one bathing-room in this building, which is particularly styled the *Kaisersbad*; it is a very elegant room, with a high, domed ceiling, the walls being lined with black and white marble; the bathing-tub is also of marble. A very elegantly fitted up anteroom for dressing is attached to the bathing-room. A small extra fee is charged for the use of this superb little *Kaisersbad*.

All the other bathing-houses likewise have excellent arrangements and furnished rooms for the accommodation of patients. The attendants are very well trained; those who do the shampooing and kneading, which is performed in a perfect manner, are called *doucheurs* or *frotteurs*.

The most important of the numerous wells is the *Kaiserquelle*, which supplies the *Kaiserbad*, *Neubad*, *Königin v. Ungarn*, and the *Elisabeth-Brunnen*. Three other wells, called *Quirinusquelle*, *Rosenquelle*, and *Corneliusquelle*, furnish the water for the other bathing-houses.

Hotels: Grand Monarque, Hotel Nuellens, Hôtel de l'Empereur, Dragon d'ôr, Dubik, Fügels Hôtel, Union Hotel.

Physicians: All practitioners in Aachen practise the bath treatment.

Access: From Hamburg or Bremen, *viâ* Cologne to Aachen; from London, to Calais or Ostend, and *viâ* Brussels, Verviers to Aachen; from Paris, *viâ* Namur, Lüttich (Liege) to Aachen.

In close proximity to Aachen is another spa, celebrated by the high temperature of its sulphur springs. This is *Burtscheid*, a city of 10,000 inhabitants. It has twenty-five thermal springs, one of which, the *Mühlenbendquelle*, is the hottest spring of central Europe (160° F.), being even hotter than the Karlsbad Sprudel. But the water contains less sulphur than that of Aachen. The climate is very healthy, and the arrangements are similar to those of Aachen. It has ten bathing-houses; the largest and best arranged hotels and bathing establishments are the *Rosenbad*, with one hundred rooms for patients, eighty bathing-rooms, and a fine garden; and the *Karlsbad*, with fifty-six furnished rooms, and sixteen bathing-rooms.

A *Kurgarten*, opposite to the Rosenbad, with pleasant walks and resting-places, is a great accommodation for invalids residing at Burtscheid. A *Trinkhalle* (fountain-hall), where patients drink the water of the *Victoriaquelle*, is in the Kurgarten.

Travelling further southward on the left bank of the Rhine, we reach the railway station, Remagen, and thence by stage,

NEUENAHR, a small village, with four hundred inhabitants, in the Ahr valley, 270 feet above the sea. Though it has existed only for a short time as a spa (since 1856), it has already become very popular. It has a mild, pure air, without sudden changes of temperature, being protected against sharp winds by high hills. The springs and hotels are on the right bank of the river Ahr. All arrangements are on a moderate scale. There is a *Kurhaus*, with a large number of furnished rooms, and a reading-room, where the following English papers can be read: London *Times*, *Galignani's Messenger*, *Illustrated London News*. The bathing-house contains forty-five bathing-rooms and appliances of all kinds of douches, as lateral, circular, ascending, stomach, uterus douches. By a five minutes' walk we reach the *Kurpark*, whose shady walks and pleasant promenades are the best features of the spa. There is a small pavilion, where patients drink the mineral water, and a long covered passage, a very primitive structure of wood and bricks, affords some shelter on rainy days. A short distance from thence is *Grosse Sprudel*, the principal spring of Neuenahr, which breaks forth with a noisy, bubbling sound, but does not ascend, as does the Karlsbad Sprudel, nor is its temperature as high as that of the latter.

Hotels: Kurhaus, Rheinischer Hof, Victoria.

Physicians: Drs. Schnitz, Feltyen, Unschuld, Stiege, Münzel, Schmidt, Mermagen, Tesehemacher.

Access: From Bremen or Hamburg, *viâ* Cologne and Bonn, to station Remagen (on the Rhine); from London, *viâ* Calais or Ostend to Brussels, Cologne, and Remagen; from Paris, *viâ* Cologne to Remagen, thence by post-omnibus or carriage to Neuenahr.

South of Neuenahr, near the river Mosel, is the little spa,

BERTRICH, a very suitable place for patients fond of a quiet but social living, and moderate prices. It is very pleasantly situated in the valley of the Mosel, between Coblenz and Trier (Treves), 433 feet above the sea; the climate is mild. Bertrich is called a *mild* Karlsbad, as its water does not contain so much sulphate of soda as the Karlsbad springs, nor has it so high a temperature. All arrangements are good and comfortable.

Hotels: Klering, Werling, Thomas, Schmidt, Schneider.

Physicians: Dr. Cüppers.

Access: From Cologne, *viâ* Coblenz to Bullay; from Paris, *viâ* Diedenhofen (Thionville) and Trier (Treves) to Bullay, thence by stage to Bertrich.

Travelling further south on the left bank of the Rhine we reach

KREUZNACH, the Mecca of all scrofulous patients,

situated in the valley of the Nahe, 330 feet above the sea, a city with 14,000 inhabitants. It is surrounded by magnificent vineyards, and is one of the warmest watering places of Germany, with a mean temperature of 73° F. The climate is healthy and very mild, though sometimes a strong breeze prevails. Kreuznach ranks foremost of all saline baths; it is the panacea of all scrofulous persons, and during the summer a place of pilgrimage for 6000 invalids. The excellent results achieved by the Kreuznach waters in the cure of scrofula are due not only to the efficacy of the water and the mild climate, but chiefly to the practical and elaborate method of treatment, and the perfect arrangements for bathing and drinking. The principal establishments are on an island, formed by two branches of the river Nahe. Here we find most of the hotels and private houses of the spa, nearly all of them surrounded by fine gardens, and built and fitted up solely for the accommodation of patients, *every house being provided with bathing-rooms*. Spa Kreuznach is a quiet, pleasant place, and the large number of gardens around the dwellings give it a very charming appearance. A wide street, adorned on each side by fine private dwellings, leads to the *Kurhaus*, which is located at the southern end of the island. It is a handsome building, with a large *salon* used as a concert-hall and dining-room, and two reading-rooms, where I found the following English newspapers:—London *Times*, *Illustrated London News*, *Daily News*, *Standard*, *Saturday Review*, *Galignani's Messenger*, *American Register*. A large terrace, 280 feet long, is added to the *Kurhaus*, and here patients enjoy their coffee, tea, &c., while listening to the music performed by the band in an elegant pavilion facing the terrace. In close proximity to the Kurhaus is an elegant iron *Trinkhalle* (fountain hall), the rendezvous of the patients who drink the salty water of the *Elisenbrunnen*. This spring issues from a hole, which is sunk forty-six feet deep into the porphyry rock. The Trinkhalle is a new structure, and has only lately been thrown open to the public.

The *Kurhaus* contains twenty-seven bathing-rooms, a fine inhalation-room for inhaling atomized saline water, and Turkish and Russian baths.

Numerous pleasant *excursions* can be made in the environs. The following points are the most favoured:—

Schlossberg (480 feet), Kuhberg, Mönchsberg, Gans (1000 feet) with a splendid view of the whole surroundings, Rheingrafenstein (700 feet), Ebernburg, once the castle of the celebrated Franz v. Sickingen.

Hotels: Visitors who stop at the railway station of the city of Kreuznach, can remain at one of the city hotels until they have hired rooms for the season at the spa; but it is more practical to leave the railway at station *Bad-Kreuznach*, and stop at one of the hotels of the spa until arrangements have been made for the whole time of the course, which generally extends to *six weeks*. Patients can make arrangements for board at most of the private houses.

Hotels (1) in the city: Pfälzer Hof, Adler, Berliner Hof; (2) in Bad-Kreuznach: Kurhaus, Oranienhof, Kauzenberg, Hôtel de l'Europe, Hôtel du Nord, Hôtel Royal, Englischer Hof.

Physicians: Drs. Michels, Priczer, Stabel, Karst, Hessel, Fleussner, Strahl, Jung, &c.

Access: From Cologne, *viâ* Coblenz, Bingen, to Kreuznach, by railway; or by steamboat on the Rhine from Cologne to Bingerbruck, thence by railway to Kreuznach; from Paris, *viâ* Metz and Saarbrück to Kreuznach.

In close proximity to Kreuznach (half-an-hour distant) is the little spa—

MÜNSTER AM STEIN, beautifully situated in a valley surrounded by steep hills, with a pure, bracing air and a mild climate; its wells and bathing arrangements are similar to those of Kreuznach. Those who prefer a quiet, cheap, and country-like place, would do well to resort thither.

Hotels: Kurhaus, Victoria, Adler, Stolzenfels, &c.

Physicians: Drs. Wilsoh, Glacssgen, and the physicians of Kreuznach.

Access: Railway from Kreuznach to Münster.

Crossing to the other side of the Rhine, we come to the most distinguished and frequented watering places of Europe, famous for luxury and high style of living, and at one time most notorious and attractive to the fashionable world by the gambling-tables, which, fortunately, have been closed since the foundation of the new German Empire. These are the Rhenish spas (popularly so-styled on account of the neighbourhood of the Rhine), of which the largest is—

WIESBADEN, the most frequented bath of Germany,

visited annually by more than 60,000 persons; it has 43,700 inhabitants. A large number of villa houses surrounded by handsome gardens present a fine appearance. Situated on the southern slope of the Taunus mountains, 323 feet above the sea, in a pleasant valley, open only towards the south and southeast, it has a very mild and warm climate, for which reason many foreigners prefer to live there during the winter. In summer it is sometimes very warm and close, and then not suitable for invalids requiring a tonic, bracing air. Wiesbaden, the capital of the former Duchy of Nassau, has all the attractions of a large, wealthy city; all arrangements are first-class, the environs very pleasing, and the proximity of the Rhine lends another charm to the spa.

Entering the city from the railway station, and turning to the right, we promenade through the *Wilhelmsstrasse*, a long, wide street with several rows of old shady trees, at the end of which we arrive at a large square, which indeed is unique. The fine garden, and the shady promenade with time-honoured chestnut-trees, the two large ponds, each with a grand fountain in the centre, the long colonnades on both sides of the square with their brilliant shops, and the magnificent *Kurhaus* in the background—all this presents a most striking appearance. And in the evening, when garden, colonnades, and Kurhaus are lighted up by an immense number of gas-lights; when the gushing waters fall over hundreds of gas-jets—placed around the fountains, and throwing their brilliant light through the glistening spray—the sight is fascinating. The colonnades, built in Doric style, are very spacious, and patients as well as sightseers throng there, eager to spend their money for the various articles exhibited attractively in the shops, the *bazaar* of Wiesbaden. But the centre of attraction to visitors is the magnificent *Kurhaus*, especially the grand concert-hall, 130 feet long, 60 feet wide, and 50 feet high, with large galleries, resting on 28 Corinthian columns, of red marble with gilded capitals. All the other *salons* are also fitted up in elegant, luxurious style; the reading-rooms contain a very large number of newspapers (English and American journals included). Added to the rear of the Kurhaus is a splendid piazza, which faces a large square planted with old trees, and adorned with a large number of orange-trees. A beautiful lake, on which graceful swans enjoy an undisturbed *dolce far niente*, completes the charming scene. This lovely spot is the afternoon rendezvous of the mass of visitors who are desirous of enjoying an hour of sweet idleness, while sipping aromatic coffee, and listening to the music performed by an excellent band.

An extensive *Kurpark*, with ponds, flower-beds, old trees, and shady walks, adjoins the *Kurhaus*, enticing patients and visitors to ramble over the delightful promenades and inhale the pure mild air. No wonder that Wiesbaden attracts many thousand visitors.

Opposite to the *Kurgarten* is the theatre, and in front of it a small square, where the bust of Schiller, the great German poet, is placed on a fine granite pedestal. A short distance from this square we enter a very long passage, covered by a neat iron structure, which leads to the *Kochbrunnen*, the most favoured of the twenty-nine springs of Wiesbaden, and for a long time the only one used for drinking. Patients here congregate in the morning, the unpleasant task of drinking the salty liquid being alleviated by the merry tunes of a lively waltz or a spirited march.

A new fountain, inclosed by a costly structure of serpentine, has just been opened (June, 1879); the name of it is *Schützenhofquelle* (107° F.)

There are thirty-two bathing establishments with 900 bathing-rooms, all the large hotels being provided with elegant baths.

Many pleasant *excursions* can be made in the neighbourhood of Wiesbaden; I mention as points of interest, Dietenmühle, Sonnenberg, Russian chapel, Platte, temple on the Neroberg.

Hotels: Nassauer Hof, Hotel Victoria, Adler, Rose, Grand Hôtel, Hôtel du Nord, Taunus Hotel, Hotel Vagel.

Physicians: Wiesbaden has a large number of experienced physicians, who all practise as bath doctors. I mention Drs. Albert, Alefeld, Bickel, Kohn, Diesterwey, Fritze, Graefe, Haas, Hartmann, Roth, Velten, &c., &c.

Access: From Bremen or Hamburg, *viâ* Cologne by railway to Wiesbaden, or from Cologne by steamboat; from London, *viâ* Cologne; from Paris, *viâ* Frankfort-on-the-Main to Wiesbaden.

After a pleasant stage ride of two and half hours from Wiesbaden, we arrive at one of the most popular iron baths—

SCHWALBACH (or Langenschwalbach), much frequented by English and Americans, 900 feet above the sea, in a narrow valley, surrounded by woods; it has 3000 inhabitants. Prices are high, and rooms are often very scarce in the height of the season (July). The powerful iron waters, combined with a pure, fresh air, are very effective in the cure of feeble and anæmic persons. All arrangements are first class. A magnificent new *Kurhaus* has just been completed (June, 1879); it contains a superb concert-hall, adorned with twenty pilasters of black marble, a large, elegant dining-*salon*, and a reading-room with the following newspapers: London *Times, Daily News, Standard, Galignani's Messenger, New York Herald.* The bathing-house has ninety bathing-rooms, all neatly fitted up, and provided with bathing-tubs of brass. On the second floor of this building, is a more elegant bathing-room, with a nicely fitted up anteroom; this is called the *prince's bath* (*Fürstenbad*), and can be used by every patient who pays the moderate fee of six marks. A large wooden building, called *Trinkhalle*, part of which is occupied by a limited number of modest-looking shops, is used for promenading on rainy days. The *Weinbrunnen*, the most popular of Schwalbach's springs, is nearly covered by a new iron pavilion; a little farther off, in the park, is the *Stahlbrunnen*. On the whole the little city looks very neat, and the large number of stately hotels and lodging-houses bear testimony of the prosperity of the place. About 5000 patients visit it annually, and 50,000 baths are given.

Excursions are made to the Paulinenberg, Ratte (1300 feet), Adolfseck, Hohenstein, &c.

Hotels: Herzog von Nassau, Post, Hôtel Métropole, Russischer Hof, Hotel Wagener, Taunus Hotel.

Physicians: Drs. Birnbaum, Böhm, Frickhöffer, Fritze, Genth, Gosebruch, Grebert.

Access: By stage from Wiesbaden.

By an hour's stage drive on a fine, shady road, we reach—

SCHLANGENBAD, the most popular spa for diseases of the nervous system and female disorders. It is a lovely little place, with 350 inhabitants, delightfully situated in a valley on the southern slope of the Taunus mountains, surrounded by high wooded hills, which afford sufficient shelter from sudden changes of temperature. Though 925 feet above the sea, it has a mild climate. The air is exceedingly pure and fresh, and acts highly beneficially on nervous persons, who resort to the little spa mostly for a stay during the whole summer. The society which congregates here is very refined, and even of an aristocratic character. The whole place looks very neat and charming, quiet and attractive. The shady promenades which surround it enjoy a great, and indeed well deserved, reputation ; there is hardly any other spa where so much attention and skill is devoted to that important requisite of a well-arranged watering place. Nature favours this bath very much, as the woods, which completely surround it, form one single grand park of the most beautiful beech-trees, in such close proximity to the dwellings that patients almost enter the woods as soon as they leave the house.

The bathing-houses and all other arrangements are

under the supervision of the government, which seems to control everything, even the charges of the washerwomen, there being a price-list posted on a wall of the Kurhaus, stating the price for washing shirts, collars, ladies' underwear, &c., and signed by the burgomaster.

The *Kurhaus* is a very modest-looking building, containing a *salon* for *réunions*, a billiard and reading-room (London *Times*, *Galignani's Messenger*). The new Trinkhalle (completed June, 1879) is a very handsome iron structure, 270 feet long. The three bathing-houses contain fifty spacious bathing-rooms, and a large number of furnished rooms for the accommodation of visitors; the number of these is 2000 annually. All the houses of the spa also have arrangements for patients.

Hotels: Nassauer Hof, Victoria, Pariser Hof, Germania.

Physicians: Drs. Bertrand, Baumann, Walf.

Access: From Cologne, by railway to station Eltville, thence by an hour's stage ride to Schlangenbad; or by railway to Wiesbaden, thence by stage (three and a half hours) to Schlangenbad.

By three hours' railway travel from Wiesbaden, on the right bank of the Rhine, we reach—

EMS, the *gem* of the German spas, and likewise one of those celebrated and luxurious Rhenish spas where all public buildings are erected and fitted up in elegant style. The streets and promenades are thronged during the season by 13,000 patients; and persons fond of seeing high life and fashionable

EMS.

Page 68.

society can there fully gratify their desire. Ems is situated in the small, picturesque valley of the Lahn, 291 feet above the sea; it has 5500 inhabitants. Being sheltered by high wooded hills from the cool north and east winds, it has a mild climate; but it cannot be denied that during the summer the heat at times is very oppressive, the temperature rising as high as 100°. Ems is a captivating place, but not a very cheap one. Beautiful environs, the close proximity of the Rhine, the completeness of all arrangements for bathing as well as for amusements, the refined society which congregates there, are attractions not often found combined. Its wells having the reputation of possessing great curative effect in cases of sterility, it is since many years the favourite watering place of the ladies. In the afternoon the *élite* of the society assembles in the *Kurgarten*, to listen to the usual afternoon concerts; in the morning the guests crowd in the *Kurhaus* at the principal springs: the *Kesselbrunnen*, *Kaiserbrunnen*, and the world-renowned *Kränchen*.

The *Kurhaus* is a large old-fashioned building, containing, besides the mineral springs, a large number of elegant bathing-rooms; in one wing some bathing-rooms, nicely fitted up, are reserved for ladies; in one of these is the far-famed *Bubenquelle* (Boys'-fountain), a thermal spring of 95°, ascending in the centre of the bathing tub.

Directly opposite to the *Kurhaus* is the inhalation-house, where the atomized mineral water is inhaled.

Close by the *Kurhaus* is the conversation-house, which at Ems is called *Kursaal*, a handsome building with superb *salons*, restaurant, &c. The *grand salon*, which is used for concerts, dancing and theatrical performances, is a magnificent room, with galleries supported by sixteen marble colums ; the reading-room is a very large, elegant room, covering the whole breadth of the house ; it was once the grand gambling *salon*, and is now stocked with a considerable number of newspapers. The following English papers are on the list : London *Times*, *Daily News*, *Telegraph*, *Galignani's Messenger*, *American Register*, *New York Herald.*

A very fine iron structure, called *Trinkhalle*, adjoins the *Kursaal;* it is a long covered walk, used for promenading on rainy days. In front of the *Kursaal* is the *Kurgarten*, and a long row of brilliant shops, the *bazaar* of Ems. Fine pleasure-grounds adjoining the Trinkhalle, shady promenades on both sides of the river Lahn, and pretty villa houses, enhance the delightful picture which the lovely little spa presents to the eyes of the tourist.

Opposite to the *Kurgarten*, on the other side of the river, is the new royal bathing-house with excellent arrangements. It contains forty-six bathing-rooms with tubs of fine white porcelain. One of these rooms, with an elegantly furnished anteroom and a marble bathing-tub, is denominated *Kaiserbad* (imperial bath), and can be used by every patient who is inclined to pay the small fee of three marks. An inhalation-room is also in the building. There are also seventeen bathing-rooms reserved for ladies exclusively, each of them provided with two separate tanks, which furnish the water for the powerful uterusdouchet, applied for disorders of the uterine system. Immense reservoirs, where the thermal water is cooled to the proper temperature, supply the baths. There is also another royal bathing-house, the *Fürstenthums*. All the government buildings contain 127 bathing-rooms. There are also several private bathing-houses with elegant arrangements.

There are many interesting and easily accessible points in the environs of Ems, with good restaurants and cafés; most of them afford a splendid view of the valley of the Rhine, the Taunus mountains, &c. The following may be mentioned: Mahlbergskopf, Bäderlei, Mooshütte, Schöne Aussicht.

Hotels: Englischer Hof, Russischer Hof, Darmstädter Hof, Hotel Guttenberg, Hotel Johannisberg, Hôtel de France.

Physicians: Drs. Cohn, Döring, Gusse, Goltz, Guttentag, Grossmann, Hill, Lange, Nalda, Orth, Panthel, Vogler, Wenkenbach, Wuth.

Access: From Bremen or Hamburg, *viâ* Cologne and Coblenz, to Ems; from London and Paris, also *viâ* Cologne, Coblenz, to Ems.

Starting from Wiesbaden, we reach by half an hour's railway ride, station *Flörsheim*, and thence by stage in twenty minutes—

WEILBACH, a sulphur spa, situated 420 feet above the sea, in an open plain on the southern slope of the Taunus mountains. It is a quiet little spot, without special attractions except the fine *Kurpark;* all arrangements are on a very small scale. There is a new bathing-house, with twelve bathing-rooms and a very fine inhalation-room, where patients inhale the sulphuretted hydrogen emanating from the sulphur water, which falls down from a high fountain. One hundred thousand bottles of sulphur water are annually exported. A lithia spring is a good adjuvant to the sulphur water.

Hotels: Vier Jahreszeiten, and Kurhaus.
Physicians: Drs. Neuroth, Stifft.

There is another spa, of far greater importance, in this neighbourhood, viz. :—

SODEN, a small city with 1500 inhabitants, very pleasantly situated, 440 feet above the sea, in a long wooded valley, at the foot of the Taunus mountains, well protected against north and east winds. It has a very mild, sedative air, which is moderately moist, and rich in ozone; there are no sudden changes of temperature. Soden has a fine *Kurgarten;* but though an old spa, it is still in want of the inevitable *Kurhaus*, although a private hotel assumes that proud name. However, there is a new bathing-house with thirty-two bathing-rooms, and with a fine pleasure-ground in front of it. An iron spring is in the immediate neighbourhood at the village of *Nauenhain.* About 3000 persons, affected chiefly with diseases of the throat and bronchial tubes, visit the place during the season.

There are pleasant *excursions* to the three Linden, Altenhamer Thal, Sulzbach, &c.

Hotels: Kurhaus, Europäischer Hof, Frankfurter Hof, Hotel Uhrig.

Physicians: Drs. Bröking, Fresenius, Köhler, Pagenstecher, Thilenius, Stöltzing, Schlüter.

Access: From Frankfort-on-the-Main by railway in thirty minutes.

We are now about to visit the once most fashionable and stylish of all the so-called Rhenish baths, which for a long time had gained the greatest notoriety by the grandeur and elegance of its establishments, and last but not least by its far-famed gambling-tables, which at present are closed. This is—

HOMBURG. Scarcely known before 1840, it has, by the aid of the gambling-tables, become one of the most frequented spas in Europe, being still visited annually by 10,000 patients and an equal number of tourists, English and Americans rushing thither in large numbers. It is pleasantly situated, 600 feet above the sea, on the slope of a hill of the Taunus mountains, well sheltered from the north and east; its 8000 inhabitants chiefly depend on the income derived from the visitors. The grand buildings of the spa—as the Kurhaus, theatre, palm-house, &c.—which have been erected by the former proprietors of the gambling-tables, have been taken possession of (since 1872) by the city; a small fee is now collected from the visitors for the purpose of keeping them in proper condition. The fear of the good citizens of Homburg of losing the patronage of the civilized world by the abolition of gambling, has proved groundless, the place having ample attractions, owing to its charming situation, complete arrangements, and effective waters. A fashionable and more select society than formerly, now congregates there, all having these two objects in view, viz. pleasure and restoration of health.

Entering the city at the railway station, we pass through the principal street, the *Louisenstrasse*, and stop at the *Kurhaus*, the centre of attraction to all visitors. It is perhaps the grandest establishment of the kind in Central Europe, only the conversation-houses of Wiesbaden and Baden-Baden being capable of bearing comparison with it; it has large, magnificent *salons*, elegantly and luxuriously fitted up, and richly ornamented; a superb ball-room with marble columns, a grand dining-*salon*, conversation-rooms, and two large comfortable reading-rooms, one for German, the other for foreign newspapers. The following English newspapers are on the catalogue: London *Times*, *Daily News*, *Telegraph*, *Pall Mall Gazette*, *Galignani's Messenger*, *New York Herald*, *New York Weekly Tribune*, *New York Weekly Times*. A long wide corridor adjoining the grand *salon*, and extending nearly over the whole length of the building, affords opportunity for promenading, if rain prevents active exercise in the open air.

Adjoining the Kurhaus to the north is a large terrace, covered with glass, where visitors have a beautiful view of the garden and the park; here is the rendezvous of the guests in the afternoon, where they take coffee, listening to the music and eyeing each other. Stepping down from this terrace, we enter the park, whose extensive grounds are very tastefully laid out. Beautiful flower-beds, fine old trees, shady walks kept in excellent order and alternating with green lawns, render the park as pleasant and attractive as nature and art can make it.

All springs are in the park, and most of them are

enclosed by elegant stone structures. The *Elizabeth-Brunnen*, where most of the visitors crowd in the morning, is surrounded by a very tasteful railing of red sandstone, the fountain itself being enclosed by a fine marble basin, while the whole floor around is paved with mosaic pavement. A short covered walk leads from thence to the palm-house, where palms and other tropical plants delight the eyes of the visitor. The long shady promenade adjoining this spring is thronged by the mass of visitors, English and Americans outnumbering the other nationalities (in 1878, about 3200 English, and nearly 700 Americans, were registered at Homburg); and so much English conversation is heard, that one might imagine himself to be promenading by the shady waters of an English watering place.

A bathing-house containing sixteen rooms is situated in the park, another one near the *Kurhaus;* but bathing is not much favoured at Homburg, as the internal application of the springs is necessary in order to produce beneficial effects.

Hotels: Vier Jahreszeiten, Russischer Hof, Europäischer Hof, Rheinischer Hof, Englischer Hof, Hôtel de France, Victoria.

Physicians: Drs. Becker, Dietz, Friedlich, Hitzel, Hoeber, Lommel, Weber, Will, Zimmer, Lewis (English).

Access: From Bremen or Hamburg, *viâ* Cassel and Frankfort-on-the-Main to Homburg; from London and Paris, to Frankfort-on-the-Main, thence to Homburg.

Not far from Frankfort, on the railway from that

city to Giessen, is another spa, which is becoming more and more popular. This is—

NAUHEIM, a city with 2500 inhabitants, situated 450 feet above the sea, on the north-east slope of the Taunus mountains. As a spa has existed only since 1834, but it has already acquired a great reputation by its efficacious wells and superior arrangements. It has a palatial *Kurhaus*, a relic of bygone times, when the gambling-tables attracted thousands of visitors. Passing through a magnificent vestibule, supported by Corinthian columns, we enter the grand *salon*, which in grandeur and elegance resembles those of the conversation-houses of Homburg, Wiesbaden, &c. On each side of it are spacious and elegant *salons*, which are used as sitting, dining, chess, and reading-rooms, the latter containing, among a large number of newspapers, the following English ones: London *Times, Illustrated London News, Punch.* A large *terrace*, ornamented with flowers, is added to the Kurhaus; descending from it, we stroll over the pleasure-grounds and promenades of an extensive *Kurpark.* By a short walk we reach the *Grosse Sprudel*, the most important well of Nauheim, extremely rich in carbonic acid; its water is only used for bathing. The spa has three bathing-houses, with 130 bathing-rooms, where at times 1000 baths a-day are given. There are also wooden boxes used for carbonic acid *gas baths.* A short distance from the bathing-houses is the *Kurbrunnen*, the most favoured by those who use the water internally.

Excursions: To the Johannisberg, Stadtwald, Schloss, Fiegenberg, Ruine, Münzenburg, &c.

Hotels : Hôtel de l'Europe, Bellevue. Deutscher Hof, Darmstädter Hof.

Physicians : Drs. Bencke, Bode, Erhardt, Groedel, Abéc, Scott.

Access : From Bremen or Hamburg, *viâ* Cassel and Giessen to Nauheim; from London, *viâ* Cologne, Coblenz, to Nauheim ; from Paris, *viâ* Frankfort-on-the-Main.

Travelling eastward, the next celebrated watering place we reach is—

KISSINGEN, a name well known to the reader, as the Kissingen water is sold perhaps by all druggists in all civilized countries. This spa is the Eldorado of dyspeptic English and Americans, who extensively patronize it. It is very pleasantly situated, in the valley of the Saale, 590 feet above the sea, protected against north and south-east winds by wooded hills. It has a mild climate ; the air is pure, and rich in ozone. About 10,000 invalids annually visit the city whose 3500 inhabitants seem to make a living only from the money spent by the visitors, there being apparently no other branches of industry carried on. The *Kurpark* is a very pretty little spot, with several rows of large, old, shady trees, where the patients perambulate in the morning from six till eight, drinking the ordained quantity of mineral water, and listening to the masterpieces of the great composers performed by a select band. All the springs—the celebrated *Pandur*, the far-famed Ragorzy, and the mild, sparkling *Maxbrunnen*—are in the Kurpark, covered by handsome iron structures. The water is here served by *male* attendants! it is fresh and palatable, and to drink it is rather a pleasure. It is usually taken cold; but if so ordered by the physician, it is warmed on practical appliances, in the shape of large tables heated by gas. Opposite to the springs are arcades, which afford ample opportunity for promenading on rainy days. The *conversation-house* is a handsome building, but not so grand, nor so elegant, as the one at Homburg or Wiesbaden; it has several nice *salons*, and a reading-room with a fair number of newspapers.

Kissingen is not a luxurious place, like Homburg or Baden-Baden; there is not so much display, and less extravagance, but more attention on the part of the visitors to the real duty, i.e., drinking and bathing. The arrangements for bathing are very good; the new bathing establishment, erected by a company, contains 120 bathing-rooms, more or less elegant according to the price.

There are very pleasant promenades adjoining the conversation-house and outside of the city; in fact, wherever we direct our steps, we find splendid woods and numerous shady walks. By half an hour's walk on shady promenades on the banks of the Saale, we reach the *Salinen*, where the magnificent salt spring, the *Sprudel*, breaks forth from the sandstone, at a depth of 300 feet, rising and falling periodically; it has an abundance of water and carbonic acid, and supplies the bathing-houses. A nice coffee-garden, in the immediate neighbourhood of the salines, is the afternoon rendezvous of the visitors. There are many patients who remain for several hours at the

Gradir-häuser (long structures, in which fagots are piled up, through which the salt water trickles), in order to inhale the air saturated with small particles of salt.

Hotels: Kurhaus, Russischer Hof, Hotel Kaiser, Hotel Victoria, Hôtel de Bavière, Preussischer Hof, &c.

Physicians: Drs. Bexberger, Dietz, Diruf, Erhard, Franqué, Pfriem, Sotier, Stöhr, Welsch.

Access: From London and Paris, to Frankfort-on-the-Main, thence *viâ* Schweinfurt to Kissingen; from Bremen or Hamburg, *viâ* Hanover, Cassel, Fulda, to Kissingen.

Promenading from Kissingen along the banks of the Saale, we arrive in about an hour at the little spa—

BOCKLET, a very quiet but pleasant place, with a strong chalybeate spring. Of course the arrangements are on a modest scale, but the place looks very attractive. There is a delightful little *Kurpark*, with very old trees and many resting-places, and a handsome *Trinkhalle;* woods, with pleasant, shady walks, surround the village. The small bathing establishment looks neat and clean; peat baths are in great favour. The iron water has a very refreshing taste, owing to the great quantity of carbonic acid. Lodgings can be had at the so-called *Kurhaus*.

This spa is an excellent place for those who like a quiet secluded retreat, and would certainly be far more patronized if that formidable rival, Kissingen, were not in the immediate neighbourhood.

Physician: Dr. Diruf, jun.

Access: From Kissingen by stage twice a-day.

By a five hours' stage drive we travel from Kissingen to—

BRÜCKENAU, a chalybeate spring, picturesquely situated in a pleasant valley, 915 feet above the sea, with a pure, bracing air. It has an elegant *Kurhaus*, built by King Ludwig I. of Bavaria, and is a very desirable place for those who like a cheap, country-like living. Number of visitors, 1000.

Hotels: Bairischer Hof, Post.
Physicians: Drs. Hermann, Imhof.
Access: From Hamburg or Bremen, *viâ* Cassel and Fulda, to station Iossa, thence by stage in two hours to Brückenau; from London and Paris, *viâ* Frankfort-on-the-Main to Iossa.

The trip through the second group of the German spas having been finished, a few words remain to be said of a spa which lies between the first and the second groups; this is—

WILDUNGEN, a place so highly recommended by the profession to patients affected with diseases of the urinary system, that it deserves to be more patronized by English and Americans suffering from such disorders. It is a small city in the duchy of Waldeck, with 2000 inhabitants, situated 840 feet above the sea, in a pleasant open valley, partly surrounded by wooded hills 1700 feet high. The climate is fresh, but not rough, though the evenings are cool and moist. The springs, bathing-houses, &c., are about twenty minutes distant from the place. These springs, though in great repute for several hundred years, were formerly not much patronized, owing to the poor arrangements; but since 1857, when a company took possession of them, they have become quite popular, many improvements having been made. A large lodging and bathing-house, containing eighty nicely furnished rooms and fifteen bathing-rooms, with tubs of slate or marble, affords good and comfortable accommodation, and also a very pleasant residence, owing to the nice garden in front of it, and the pleasant view of the city, mountains, valleys, &c. In close proximity, but one hundred feet higher, lies a handsome *Kurhaus*, with a large concert *salon*, dining and reading-room. By half an hour's walk we reach the most renowned of the springs, the *Helenenquelle*, situated in a ravine, surrounded by high hills. A fine, antique temple, with a handsome portico, supported by two caryatides, has been erected over the spring. The water is bright, sparkling, and very refreshing. Another much-favoured spring, the *Victorquelle*, is most pleasantly located in the wood, not far from the lodging-house. At the other end of the spa is the *Königsquelle*, the property of Dr. Rörig, and the richest in carbonic acid. A bathing-house with twelve bathing-rooms is attached to it, and a spacious garden and covered walk afford ample room for promenading. The whole place looks quiet and country-like, and is well suited to patients fond of quiet living. The number of visitors has steadily increased from 358 in 1857, to 1700 in 1875; more than 30,000 bottles of the mineral water are annually exported. The woods in the rear of the lodging-house afford shady promenades.

Excursions are made to the Zickzackberg, Homberg (1655 feet), Ratzenstein, &c.

Lodgings : The best accommodations are in the *Logirhaus* (lodging-house), others in Hôtel de Russie, Hof von Waldeck, Post.

Physicians : Drs. Rörig, Doehne, Krüger, Lingelsheim, Marc, Stoecker.

Access : From London or Paris, viâ Frankfort-on-the-Main, to station Wabern (near Cassel) ; from Bremen or Hamburg, viâ Hanover and Cassel to Wabern ; from Wabern by stage in two hours to Wildungen.

From Frankfort-on-the-Main we continue our trip in a southerly direction, to visit the third group of the German spas. They are all situated in the southern part of Germany, viz., in Baden, Würtemberg, and Bavaria. By express train from Frankfort, through one of the most charming regions of Germany, we reach in four and a half hours—

BADEN-BADEN, the *crowning glory* of all German spas. Its situation, and the completeness of all arrangements, the charming environs, and the fashionable society which assembles there every season, all unite to make a sojourn at this beautiful spot most delightful and pleasant. Therefore it is not surprising that the *élite* of the whole world resort to this little paradise, either for recreation or amusement. About 50,000 persons visit it annually Frenchmen especially were formerly accustomed to flock thither in large numbers, and gave the place quite a French appearance. French style, French manners, and French *demi-monde* prevailing more than desirable. This has somewhat changed since the last Franco-German war. Moreover, the gambling-rooms having been closed in 1872, the greatest attraction for a certain class of people has disappeared. These *habitués* of the *faro table* are now conspicuous by their absence, but their non-appearance is not complained of. English and Americans, and especially the Russian nobility, patronize the place very extensively. A large number of splendid villas, erected by aristocrats or rich nabobs, contribute materially to enhance the natural beauty of the spa. Theatre and races are attractions for many visitors.

Baden-Baden, 616 feet above the sea, has 11,000 inhabitants. Its situation on the right bank of the little rivulet Oos, in a picturesque and romantic valley at the entrance to the Black Forest, is fascinating. It is surrounded by high hills, which are covered with fine forests. Being protected by these against the cool north and east winds, it has a mild, moderately moist, and very healthy climate. The mean temperature of the year is 50°—of the winter, 35°; there are no sudden changes of temperature.

There are twenty wells, which furnish an abundance of water of 140°—154°, mainly used for bathing, the baths being given at the large hotels and in the new bathing-house called *Friedrichsbad*.

This new bathing-house is undoubtedly the grandest, most luxurious, and most perfect establishment of the kind in Germany, the most costly materials having been employed in its erection. It is most skilfully and practically planned and executed, and cannot be surpassed in point of elegance, comfort, and completeness of all arrangements. An abundance of the best Italian marble has been used for large swimming-baths and bathing-tubs, and all the rooms are painted and ornamented in the most elegant and tasteful manner. Extraordinary cleanliness prevails everywhere, and the attendance is excellent, the *Bademeister* (waiters) being well trained, and skilful in shampooing and kneading. The temperature of the various rooms is well regulated, and the heat in the Turkish and Russian baths is mild and agreeable.

The lower story of the building contains a large vestibule, supported by four columns: on each side of it are *Wildbäder*—single bathing-rooms—for cold water treatment, an inhalation-room, and an electric bath. The rooms for single baths are spacious and airy, the tubs are constructed of one single block of Italian marble, and sunk into the floor of the room; each room is provided with a douche and a shower-bath. The so-called *Wildbäder* are basins (18 feet by 10 feet), about twenty inches deep, where several persons bathe at the same time, and the warm mineral water constantly runs in and off; the floor is cemented, and covered with fine sand. Patients quietly lie on the floor during the whole time they remain in the bath, after the fashion prevailing at the spa in *Wildbad*, Würtemberg (hence the name). The adjoining rooms have comfortable beds, for patients who need rest after the bath. The room for cold-water treatment contains all kinds of douches — lateral, ascending, descending, circular douches, &c., &c., and a cold water bath (10 feet by 5 feet), the walls of which are lined lined with blue porcelain.

By a grand staircase we ascend to the second story. A lofty hall (200 feet by 26 feet) is used for promenading and as a reception-room. We now enter the most important and luxurious part of the building, namely, the large Turkish and Russian baths, swimming baths, &c., (called society baths, as a number of persons bathe together). The principal feature of these baths is the large *cupola-room*, situated directly in the centre of the building, fifty-five feet high, and beautifully constructed and frescoed; it contains the grand *circular* swimming-basin, twenty-six feet in diameter, built of Carrara marble, with circular steps leading down into the water. On each side of the cupola-room are the ladies' and the gentlemen's departments of the Turkish and Russian baths, each department containing two hot-air (Turkish) rooms, two vapour-rooms, a shampooing-room, a spacious shower-room, with a large number of douches of every shape, size, and temperature, and a cold swimming-bath, and a large oval swimming-bath (25 feet by 10 feet) of Italian marble, and filled with tepid mineral water. Large *salons*, with small apartments for dressing, and elegant reception-rooms, are adjacent to the bathing-rooms.

The third story of the building contains vapour-baths for the use of single persons; being very luxuriously fitted up, they are called princes' baths, and charged accordingly. On the same floor are also some second-class vapour-baths, for the use of persons who are not admitted to the society baths.

This brief description will give only a faint idea of the establishment, but we are not allowed to devote more time and space to the subject, however interesting it may be to the numerous visitors of the celebrated spa.

The bath life in Baden-Baden, as in all the German spas, concentrates at the conversation-house, the public gardens, and promenades. The *conversation*, or *Kurhaus*, is 370 feet long, and has a large portico, supported by eight Corinthian columns; it contains a large number of magnificent *salons*, ornamented in grand and extravagant style, the largest of these being 160 feet long and 50 feet wide. One of these elegant *salons* is set apart as a reading-room, with about 150 newspapers and periodicals from all parts of the civilized world. Close by is the *Trinkhalle*, a noble edifice 270 feet long, with a magnificent portico, supported by sixteen Corinthian columns, and with a large rotunda, in which the mineral water is served by a young girl at a costly marble fountain. Here the patients assemble in the morning—drinking, promenading, and chatting. East of the conversation house is the *bazaar*—two rows of shops, where the best fancy articles manufactured at Paris, Vienna, and Berlin are sold at high prices. When the regular concert takes place in front of the conversation-house (between 3 to 4, and 8 to 10 p.m.), the promenades there are crowded with an elegant and gay multitude, some drinking coffee or taking supper, others walking about to see and to be seen: it is a grand sight to those who are fond of seeing it. When the concerts are over, the mass of visitors throng the splendid park, and the celebrated promenade on the left bank of the Oos, called the *Lichtenthal Allée;* this is a long drive, planted with beautiful oak, linden, and maple-trees, interspersed with bosquets and fountains. The elegant carriages of the fashionable world, the numerous riders on horseback, and the immense crowd of stylishly-dressed people walking up and down, present a lively and interesting picture scarcely seen anywhere else. At the end of this drive we reach the little village *Lichtenthal*, with good restaurants, gardens, and an old monastery, inhabited by the Cistercian nuns. Near by is the *Caevilienberg*, with fine walks and splendid views.

The environs of Baden-Baden are so charming, and the places to which excursions are made, are so numerous and picturesque, that hardly any other spa can compete with this one. I mention only the old castle Hohenbaden, and the top of the Battert (1800 feet), the Ebersteinburg, Mercuriusberg (2240 feet), Ebersteinschloss, Favorite.

Hotels: Victoria Hotel, Badischer Hof, Englischer Hof, Europaeischer Hof, Russischer Hof.

Physicians: Drs. Baumgärtner, Berton, Brunen, Gans, Heiligenthal, Knecht, Lichtenauer, Müller, Schiel, Schliep, Schmidt, Schrander, Seelos, Wilhelmi, Frey.

Access: From London, *viâ* Frankfort-on-the-Main; from Paris, *viâ* Strasburg to Baden-Baden; from Bremen and Hamburg, *viâ* Hanover, Cassel, Frankfort, to Baden-Baden.

There is a very pleasant trip from Baden-Baden, *viâ*

Gernsbach (in the Black Forest) to *Wildbad;* to those who are fond of much active exercise, it is recommendable as a march of eight hours.

WILDBAD, a very popular spa, in the kingdom of Würtemberg, lies in the charming and romantic valley of the Enz, 1323 feet above the sea; it has 3000 inhabitants. The air is pure and bracing. The whole place consists of two streets, which run along the banks of the river, the valley being very narrow, and bounded on both sides by wooded heights. The principal building is the *Kurhaus*, on the right bank of the river; it is a fine edifice, built of red sandstone, and contains a large concert *salon*, restaurant, and reading-room (with the London *Daily News*), all in the upper story, while the lower part is occupied by the baths. There are four *society baths*, fifty private baths for single persons, and five elegant bathing-rooms, called *princes' baths*, for high personages, or those patients who can afford to pay a high price. These *princes' baths* are very high and airy, with a domed ceiling and coloured skylight; the bathing-tubs are round spacious excavations in the floor, lined with white porcelain. Marble steps lead down to the water. The bottom of the tub is covered with fine sand, on which the bathers repose, while the warm mineral water constantly enters from the bottom by means of pipes. In order to reach the thermal water, a number of holes are bored through the granite rocks to a depth of 100 and 150 feet. The temperature of the springs is 93° to 94°, and remains the same, no matter how deep the holes are bored. Thirty-six holes, in which iron pipes are placed, furnish the water for all the baths.

Spacious anterooms, elegantly fitted up, and provided with carpets, are attached to these *princes' baths*. There are four large common baths (*society baths, Gesellshafts-bäder*), two for ladies two for gentlemen, each of them large enough to accommodate forty persons, and much patronized by patients who are fond of chatting and gossiping while in the bath. The depth of the water being only eighteen inches, patients must lie quietly on the soft sand of the floor, reclining against the wall of the basin. These baths are also filled with the thermal water by means of pipes, which were run through the granite ground to the proper depth, until the source of the water was struck. Patients need not refrain from using these baths, as the water is constantly renewed. The private bathing-rooms are neatly fitted up, and furnished with porcelain tubs. In every room is an apparatus for heating towels and sheets.

On the whole, the arrangements are perfect, and the Government of Würtemburg, which is the owner of the baths, deserves great credit for the exemplary manner in which all arrangements are completed.

On the other side of the river, a few hundred feet distant from the Kurhaus, a large, neat, iron structure, called *Trinkhalle* (fountain-hall) has lately been erected; here those patients who believe in the efficacy of the Wildbad water when internally employed, are at liberty to drink as much of it as they choose. Fine shady walks in the rear of the *Trinkhalle* lead to the surrounding woods.

The number of visitors already exceeds 6000; about 130,000 baths are given during the season. There are nice promenades along the banks of the Enz, and quite a number of pleasant excursions to the Black Forest afford ample opportunity for active exercise.

Hotels: Badhotel, Bellevue, Bär, Hotel Keim, Krone.

Physicians: Drs. Renz, Burkhard, Schönleber, Haussman sen. and jun.

Access: From London, *viâ* Frankfort-on-the-Main and Heidelberg; from Paris, *viâ* Strasburg; from Bremen or Hamburg, *viâ* Cassel, Frankfort, Heidelberg to Wildbad.

By a four hours' railway ride from Wildbad we reach Stuttgart, the capital of the kingdom of Würtemberg, and close by is the spa—

CANNSTADT, a city with 7000 inhabitants, 600 feet above the sea. Owing to its mild climate it has already attained some reputation as a climatic health resort. It has fourteen wells, which supply a large number of bathing establishments. The arrangements are good, though on a small scale compared with those of the spas near the Rhine. There is a neat *Kursaal*, a long brick building, nicely frescoed, for promenading on rainy days. The establishment of Dr. Veiel for the cure of skin diseases, and Dr. Ebner's orthopædic institute, enjoy a great and well-deserved reputation. As there are always so many American families who temporarily reside at Stuttgart, I consider it proper to draw their attention to a watering place so near by, which has such good and comfortable arrangements. Cannstadt has also a large number of excellent boarding-schools.

The road from Stuttgart to Cannstadt, through the

park (called *Schlossgarten*) is a most magnificent promenade. Several royal palaces, with beautiful gardens, and fine walks, picture-galleries, &c., are in the immediate vicinity.

Hotels: Hotel Herrman, Wilhelmsbad (with a good Russian and Turkish bath), Hotel Burger, Merz.

Physicians: Drs. Kiel, Tritschler sen. and jun., Wadelin, Rühle.

Access: The same as to Wildbad.

A place of great reputation, whose springs are very efficacious in cases of bronchial affections, and which is very easily accessible to English and Americans visiting Munich, is—

REICHENHALL, about three and a half hours from Munich, by the Munich-Salzburg railway. It is very picturesquely situated in the Bavarian Alps, 1407 feet above the sea, surrounded on three sides by high mountains, of 4500 feet and 6000 feet elevation; it is a small city with 3200 inhabitants. All arrangements are good, on a moderate scale, with moderate prices. There is the *Kurhaus Achselmanstein* with a fine garden, and opposite to it the *Gradirhaus*, where the strong salt water evaporates, the patients inhaling the air saturated with the small particles of salt; the new park close by is very handsome. Although spa Reichenhall has not been longer than thirty years in existence, it is already one of the most popular of the German saline baths, being visited annually by nearly 5000 patients. The air is very pure and invigorating, the mean temperature 64°. The treatment is much aided by the inhalation of compressed air, by whey and milk cures, peat baths, &c. The saline works of Reichenhall are the grandest of all in Germany. Fifteen strong salt springs issue from the earth at a depth of eighty feet, supplying not only the Reichenhall establishments, but also by pipes of several miles' length, the baths at Rosenheim, Traunstein, and Kreuth.

Visitors should not forget to visit the *Saline*, and to step down to the places where the springs break forth.

There is much opportunity for pleasant excursions in the neighbourhood; everywhere the scenery is highly interesting and romantic. The beautiful city of *Salzburg* is reached in one hour by railway; *Berchtesgaden* in two and a half hours by stage; thence, by a short promenade of one and a half hour, we reached the celebrated *Königssee*, the most romantic, perhaps, of all Alpine lakes.

Hotels: Kurhaus Achselmannstein, Louisenbad, Marienbad, Maximiliansbad, Bad Kirchberg, Hotel Burkert, Post, &c.

Physicians: Drs. v. Liebig, Geeböck, Schneider, Camerer, Rapp, Pachmeyer, Bergson, Solger, Schmidt, Kramer, Burdach.

Access: From London, *viâ* Frankfort and Munich; from Paris, *viâ* Strasburg, Stuttgart, and Munich; from Bremen and Hamburg, *viâ* Munich to Reichenhall.

There is another Alpine bath in the Bavarian Alps, which deserves to be noticed, and recommended to those who prefer a quiet, secluded place, refined society, and high Alpine region. Such a place is—

Kreuth, 2910 feet above the sea; it is a beautiful, lonely spot, surrounded by steep mountains, with a pure, fresh, and moist air. There are no other houses than the buildings for bathing and boarding, which present a very fine appearance; in fact everything looks neat and pleasant, and prices for board are very moderate. The place is much patronized by a good class of people, but for a prolonged stay it is apt to become dull to English and Americans. It has come into great reputation by its excellent wheys, which are not surpassed by the best wheys of Switzerland. Salt baths are given, the brine being carried up from Rosenheim and Reichenhall. The mountain bitters, prepared from herbs growing on the surrounding mountains, are very much praised and used. Persons affected with bronchial diseases are the patrons of Kreuth.

Those fond of excursions may visit the charming *Tegernsee* and the romantic *Achensee*.

Physicians: Drs. Beetz, Stephan.

Access: From Munich, by railway, *viâ* Holzkirchen, to station Schaftlach (one and a half mile), thence by stage in three and a half hours to Kreuth.

SILESIA.

The *fourth* group of German spas embraces the Silesian watering places, situated in the Prussian province. They are scarcely known to English and Americans, that region being really a *terra incognita* to English and American tourists. Still the *Riesengebirge* (Giant Mountains) deserve to be visited by them, owing to their picturesque scenery, and the plain good living in this part of Germany, which, it cannot be denied, is a little out of the route of the vast crowd of tourists ; this perhaps is the reason why I have not met any English or Americans in these mountains.

However, as many of these reside at Berlin, or Dresden, and some may be advised to visit one of the Silesian spas, which are easily reached by railway from these cities, I shall mention for their information those places which have the most efficacious wells and enjoy the greatest popularity. The arrangements are generally good, but on a small scale compared to the great spas in Western Germany; prices are moderate enough, though not so low as many might expect them to be in a part of the country which is so little favoured by the majority of tourists and invalids. These baths have the advantage of a plain bath-life and good society ; there is no display, no elegance, and no extravagance, as there is at the Rhenish baths ; they are frequented almost exclusively by the middle classes of North Germany. The most popular of these spas is—

OBERSALZBRUNN, or Salzbrunn, a small city with 5800 inhabitants, situated 1200 feet above the sea, in romantic valley, surrounded by hills, but open to the north-west. The air is tonic and invigorating, but there are cold winds and sudden changes of temperature. Excellent wheys are prepared. There are nice promenades, and plenty of opportunity is offered for pleasant excursions. Number of visitors about 3000.

Hotels: Flammender Stern, Krone, Brunnenhof, Sonne, Kurhaus.

Physicians : Drs. Biefel, Hoffmann, Straehler, Stempelmann, Valentiner.

Access: From Dresden or Berlin, *viâ* Görlitz to station Salzbrunn.

By a three and a half hours' ride on the Silesian mountain railway, we travel from Salzbrunn to Hirschberg; by a further ride of one and a half hours by stage we reach—

WARMBRUNN, next to Salzbrunn the most popular of the Silesian spas. It is a small place with 2500 inhabitants, situated 1100 feet above the sea, near the northern slope of the Riesengebirge; the air is invigorating, but at times a little rough. The arrangements are good; there is a handsome Kurhaus and a small bazaar, and quite a number of promenades. The surroundings are very pleasant, and afford much opportunity for excursions without danger of great fatigue. Warmbrunn is an excellent starting-point for a trip through the Riesengebirge. Such a tour, if made by short trips, is highly interesting and invigorating, without overtaxing the strength of invalids who are not too much debilitated.

Hotels : Hôtel de Prusse, Schwarzer Adler, Schneekoppe, Stadt London.

Physicians: Drs. Franz, Herzog, Höhne, Lange, Luchs, Nuchten.

Access: From Berlin or Dresden, *viâ* Görlitz to Hirschberg, thence by stage to Warmbrunn.

Starting from Salzbrunn in a southerly direction, we reach by a two and a half hours' railway ride the city of Glatz; thence after a three hours' stage drive, we arrive at—

LANDECK, a sulphur bath, 1389 feet above the sea, in a very romantic valley of the Glatz Mountains. The climate, though a mountain climate, is mild and invigorating, the north and east winds being kept off by the mountains. There are two large common baths immediately over the springs, and forty single baths. Wheys and mountain bitters are also prescribed. About 3000 patients annually visit the spa. It has a splendid park, and excellent opportunity for quite a number of excursions into the picturesque Glatz Mountains.

Hotels: Löwe, Deutsches Haus, Schlössel.

Physicians: Drs. Langner, Wehse, Schütze, Joseph, Astrowicz.

Access: From Berlin or Dresden, *viâ* Görlitz and Konigszelt to Glatz, thence by stage to Landeck.

West of Glatz are two other baths, which are very popular, both situated in the Glatz Mountains, *Reinerz* and *Cudorva*.

REINERZ, 1700 feet above the sea, in a charming valley, has the reputation of enjoying immunity from tubercular affections. The air is pure, but sudden changes of temperature often occur. The bathing arrangements are very good, the promenades and environs very fine. About 2600 visitors congregate there every season.

Hotels: Bär, Deutsches Haus.

Physicians: Drs. Berg, Drescher, Secchi, Kolbe, Zdralek.

Access: From Berlin or Dresden, to Glatz, thence by stage in two hours to Reinerz.

CUDOWA, 1235 feet above the sea, on the southern slope of the Heuschauer Mountains (2900 feet), not far from the railway station Nachod, is a small place with 700 inhabitants. The climate, though mild, is tonic and invigorating. It has nice promenades and good arrangements for bathing; there is a new establishment for peat baths, and a new and excellent Russian vapour bath. The place is becoming popular, the number of visitors already amounting to 1200 annually

Hotels: Waidmannsruh, Stern, Sonne, Neue Welt.
Physicians: Drs. Scholz, Jacob.
Access: From Dresden or Berlin, *viâ* Görlitz and Ruhbauk to station Nachod, thence by stage to Cudowa.

APPENDIX.

There are several large cities in Germany which have been often mentioned in the preceding chapter as starting-points to the various watering places, viz: Bremen, Hamburg, Cologne, Frankfort-on-the-Main, Munich, Dresden, Berlin. English and Americans arriving at one or the other of these cities, and desirous of taking a short rest, may wish to know the names of some hotels. For the information of those not in possession of a travelling guide, I shall give the names of those hotels which Baedeker, the most reliable of all guides, has marked as the best in his guide-books.

Bremen: Hillmann's Hotel, Hôtel de l'Europe, Grand Hôtel du Nord, Stadt Frankfurt, Hotel Kiedenburg.

Hamburg: Hôtel de l'Europe, Streit's Hotel, Victoria Hotel, Kronprinz, Hotel St. Petersburg, Alster Hotel, Zing's Hotel, Hoefer's Hotel.

Cologne: Hôtel du Nord, Hotel Disch, Mainzer Hof, Pariser Hof, Wiener Hof, Victoria Hotel, Hôtel St. Paul, Hôtel Ernst.

Frankfort-on-the-Main: Frankfurter Hof, Russischer Hof, Englischer Hof, Brüsseler Hof, Landsburg.

Munich: Vier Jahreszeiten, Bayrischer Hof, Hôtel Bellevue, Hotel Detzer, Englischer Hof, Rheinischer Hof.

Dresden: Hôtel Bellevue, Victoria Hotel, Hôtel de Saxe, Kronprinz, Stadt Wien, Grand Union-Hôtel, Stadt Berlin, Stadt Gotha, Weber's Hotel.

Berlin: Kaiserhof, Hôtel Royal, Meinhardt's Hotel, Hôtel du Nord, Hôtel de Rome, British Hotel, Hôtel d'Angleterre, Hôtel de Russie.

CHAPTER II.

THE WATERING PLACES OF AUSTRIA.

THE German provinces of the Austrian Empire have an abundance of very efficacious mineral springs, especially Bohemia, Salzburg, and Styria. Some of these waters, as those of Karlsbad and Teplitz, have for hundreds of years enjoyed a world-wide reputation, and are visited by large numbers of patients from all parts of the globe; while others, less reputed, are mainly patronized by Austrians and Germans, and some almost exclusively by Austrians. All these spas are well managed, their bathing arrangements generally being even preferable to those of many German spas. The bathing-rooms are quite elegant, the tubs being mostly of marble, porcelain, or stone; the attendants are everywhere very well trained, and very accommodating, and are easily satisfied with a small *Trinkgeld* (gratuity); even at most of the common (society) baths, where only a small fee is charged, patients on coming from the bathing-room are very carefully rubbed off with towels and sheets, warmed on a large stove.

There is no such display of style as at the Rhenish spas, not even at Karlsbad or Ischl, the most fashionable of the Austrian baths. Even at these, we do not find the extravagance or the high life of Baden-Baden or Homburg. But there is an excellent tone at most of the Austrian spas, and generally we meet a very good society, especially at the smaller ones. The inhabitants are complaisant and obliging; food and drink, a very important matter in the eyes of every Austrian, are everywhere well prepared, and *first-class* at all the better hotels and restaurants. Accommodations in hotels and lodging-houses are comfortable, though perhaps not so elegant and complete as at the great German spas. Strangers travelling in Austria, feel far more comfortable and better pleased than anywhere else; this, at least, is my experience, after having travelled in Austria so many years, and having conversed with so many patients and tourists. It is really surprising that English and Americans, who are so sagacious in ferreting out pleasant and comfortable places, have so much neglected the beautiful regions of Tyrol, Salzburg, Styria, &c. More picturesque and delightful spots can scarcely be found anywhere else than in the Alpine regions of these Austrian provinces.

A patient wishing to resort to an Austrian spa, has the choice of any climate he may consider suitable for his case. He can repair to a spa with a warm, mild air, only a few hundred feet above the level of the sea; or he may betake himself to the invigorating air of an elevation of 1500 feet or 2000 feet; or to an Alpine climate of 3000 feet elevation.

We shall now commence our trip through the principal spas of *German-Austria*. They can be classified into three groups. The *first* and northern

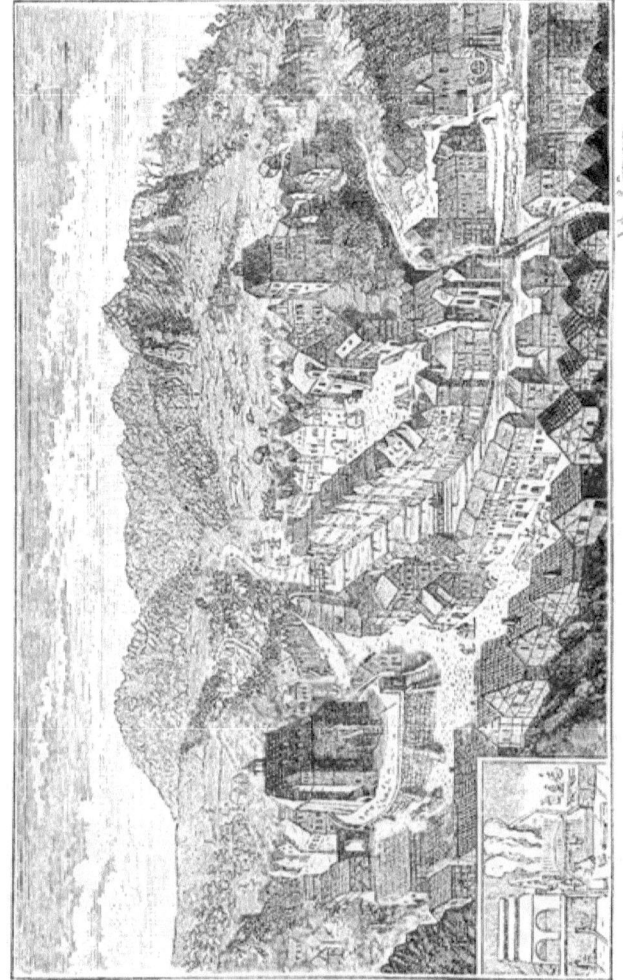

KARLSBAD.

Page 121.

group comprises the Bohemian spas: Karlsbad, Marienbad, Teplitz, Franzensbad, Johannisbad, Elster; the last-named, although situated in Saxony close to the Bohemian frontier, is generally ranked among the Bohemian spas, to which it really belongs, owing to its location and chemical properties.

The spas of the *second group* are situated in the central portion of *German-Austria* (Upper and Lower Austria and Salzburg). Baden near Vienna, Vöslau, Hull, Ischl, Aussee, and Gastein, belong to this class.

The *third group* embraces the Styrian baths: Tobelbad, Gleichenberg, Rohitsch, Tüffer, Neuhaus, Römerbad, and the little spa Villach in Kärnthen (Carinthia), all these places being located in the southern part of *German-Austria*.

1. THE BOHEMIAN SPAS.

The most celebrated and most important of these —nay, I may truly say, of all continental baths, and the one to which we shall at once direct our steps, is—

KARLSBAD, *the queen of the European spas.*

The importance of the place, and its world-wide fame, may excuse the author for devoting to its description a little more time and a larger space than to any other spa. We shall give a somewhat detailed account of the arrangements, for the benefit of English and Americans, who for some few years have extensively patronized this celebrated spa.

Karlsbad is situated in the romantic, narrow valley of the Tepel, 1200 feet above the sea (371 mètres). It is a wealthy, industrious city, with 12,000 inhabitants, and nearly 900 houses, which are built on both sides of the river: it is surrounded by high hills covered with pine and beech trees. The air is pure and salubrious; north and north-west winds prevail; the weather is variable, and rapid changes of temperature often occur. The mornings and evenings are generally very cool, even during the warmest portion of the season, the mean temperature being 43°. During the day it is often very warm and close. This spa is considered a healthy city, as it never yet has been visited by any epidemic, cholera not excepted.

Karlsbad, which is endowed with the most powerful thermal waters on the face of the globe, has existed as a watering place for more than 500 years. During the first two centuries of its existence, the waters were only used for *bathing*, ten or eleven hours of the day then being devoted to this occupation, until the skin of the patient was entirely corroded. Such a corrosion was considered the crisis, and was hailed as the return of health. In 1520, by recommendation of Dr. Payer, patients commenced to *drink* the water, and bathing gradually became so unpopular, that it was entirely abandoned in the middle of the last century. Immense quantities of water were prescribed by the bath doctors, and swallowed by the unfortunate patients. They commenced with 15 or 18 cups (about 120 ounces), increasing the number to 30, and even 40 cups (over 200 ounces) daily. The whole quantity was drunk at home, every active exercise being forbidden. This irrational treatment was abolished by the exertion of an eminent physician,

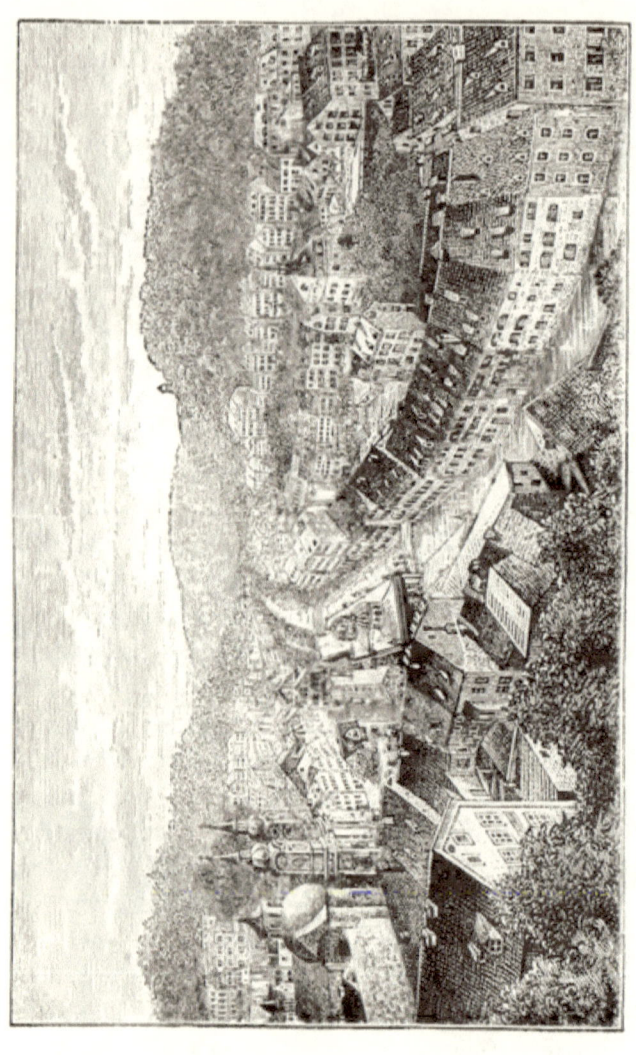

KARLSBAD.

Page 122.

Dr. Becher (1725—1792), who considerably reduced the quantity of the water, at the same time recommending patients to drink it at the wells, and to take active exercise. It was he who again advised bathing as an essential part of the cure. At the beginning of this century, it still was customary to drink from 10 to 15 cups, but gradually this number was reduced to eight and four, and even less, namely, half a cup once or twice in the morning. I am under the impression that the bath physicians sometimes go into the other extreme, i. e., of reducing the quantity of the water to a minimum, relying wholly on the diet, change of air, &c., as sufficient agencies in effecting a cure.

The official records of Karlsbad show a wonderful increase in the number of visitors since 1756, as will be seen by the following table :—

Year.	Patients.	Year.	Patients.	Year.	Patients.
1756	134	1800	744	1850	4,227
1760	162	1810	1255	1860	6,366
1770	322	1820	1461	1870	9,729
1780	225	1830	2448	1875	15,642
1790	368	1840	2882	1878	16,158

The total number of patients, and persons accompanying them, in 1875, was more than 20,000, tourists not included. These visitors came from all parts of the globe, the majority, of course, from Europe, and principally from Germany; however, America, Asia, Africa, and even Australia, are well represented on the official list. In 1877, the names of 436 Englishmen and 334 Americans were recorded as having been under medical treatment at the Karlsbad springs.

With great pride the annalists of Karlsbad enumerate the vast number of emperors, kings, princes, generals, and other celebrated personages, who have patronized that time-honoured spa; to mention them would be of no interest whatsoever to English and Americans. Only three names shall be mentioned: Goethe, Schiller, and Beethoven; these belong to mankind.

In 1844, the export of the Karlsbad mineral waters commenced; at present, over 1,000,000 quart bottles are annually sent to all parts of the world.

There is one great difference between Karlsbad and the other Bohemian baths on one side, and the Rhenish baths on the other, namely, while the latter are visited by a large number of persons seeking amusement and a luxurious life, Karlsbad is almost exclusively patronized by persons who are really suffering, and desirous of being restored to health. By some it has therefore been styled "*the* hospital of the whole civilized world," and this, in truth, it is; and a regular, thorough bath treatment at Karlsbad, is by no means a *fancy cure*. Already in 1522 Dr. Payer said, "Nature has created this bath for patients, not for anybody's lust or amusement." There is no extravagance either in amusements or fashionable display; there are no races, nor anything else that is apt to create excitement.

However, the reader should not become impressed with the idea that bath life at Karlsbad is dull, gloomy, and stern, owing to the large number of visitors who are all suffering from severe diseases; by no means. The sight of the chequered multitude, assembled from all parts of the globe, each one inspired with the hope of a speedy recovery by the aid of the far-famed springs, many having already experienced their beneficial influence; the beautiful environs, the various entertainments—all these tend to gratify the patient's mind, and to produce cheerful and hopeful feelings.

Bath life at Karlsbad is somewhat different from that at the spas hitherto described, there being really no centre of attraction in the shape of a *Kurgarten* and *Kurhaus*, situated in a convenient place. The Karlsbad *Kurhaus* is somewhat distant from the principal springs and the centre of the city; and is not surrounded by shady promenades. The thousands of patients who drink the waters are obliged to do so at the different places where the springs issue; and after having finished their morning task, they disperse to the various coffee-gardens. In the afternoon and evening concerts are given at several places, and by different bands, though those given by the *Kurcapelle*, under the able leadership of Mr. Labitzky, attract the largest audience.

The great mass of patients assemble in the morning at the *Sprudel* and the *Mühlbrunnen*, especially at the latter, the next favoured of all the springs. Here the concourse of people is really astonishing, and affords an interesting spectacle, especially to English and Americans, who eye with surprise the strange faces, and yet stranger costumes and manners, of patients coming from various climates, and of various nations. Grand new colonnades, built at an expense of half a million florins, afford shelter from rain or sun to the hundreds of invalids who, step by step, slowly advance, until the fountain is reached. These colonnades are a grand structure, but somewhat too heavy, and when many persons crowd there, the air soon becomes close. It is advisable to drink early in the morning, in order to avoid delay. The Sprudel colonnade, which, until the fall of 1878, was an old wooden structure, has lately been replaced by a grand edifice, built of iron and glass. It is a magnificent hall of immense size, and was erected during the winter of 1878-79, at an expense of 228,000 florins. Many high and richly-gilded pilasters, and a large number of exotic plants, which are placed along the walls, give a gay appearance to the interior of the hall, and delight the eyes of the hundreds of visitors who throng the place every morning, gazing with amazement at that far-famed *Sprudel*, whose boiling waters boisterously break forth from the depth of the earth, rising as high as three or four feet, ascending and descending, foaming and reeking, and throwing thick clouds of vapour up to the openings in the ceiling of the building. It is a grand sight, and many stand there admiring this grand phenomenon, and meditating upon the nature of it. The following explanation, given by Dr. Hlawaeck, the historiographer of Karlsbad, seems to be the most plausible:—" The atmospheric waters are collected at a depth of about 7000 feet, in the crevices of the granite mountain range on which the city of Karlsbad is located. The natural heat of the earth at such a depth being 167°, the waters assume the same temperature, and with the aid of a large quantity of carbonic acid, dissolve and decompose a portion of the soluble mineral constituents of the granite; saturated with these, they are raised by the pressure of the subterranean gases, and burst forth."

An extension of the Sprudel colonnade, constructed in the same style, encloses the *Hygeiensquelle*. A statue of the goddess *Hygeia* is placed in the centre of this extension building, surrounded by two beautiful palm-trees, and other exotic plants.

Near the Mühlbrunnen a large costly building has been erected, called the *Kurhaus*. It is a grand structure, but not elegant in appearance, and does not at all compare with the tasteful buildings of a similar kind at the German spas; the lower story is used for bathing purposes, the bathing-rooms being high and airy, and some of them, called *salon baths*, are fitted up with some elegance. There is also a neat reception-room on the same floor. The upper story is occupied by a large *concert salon*, restaurant, and three reading-rooms, which are liberally provided with a large number of newspapers and periodicals. Great care has been taken to supply them with a large number of English neswpapers, as the following list will demonstrate: London *Times, Standard, Punch, Illustrated London News, New York Herald, New York Tribune, American Register, Galignani's Messenger*.

Readers pay a small fee for admission.

A little farther off is another large building, the *Militair-Krankenhaus*, a hospital for soldiers of the Austrian army, and close by a fine *Kurgarten* has been laid out, and planted with a large number of trees: as this little park is yet without shade and without other attractions, patients do not much patronize it. It is intended to erect there a large elegant pavilion for concerts, which will undoubtedly render this part of the city more attractive.

The baths, which yield a large income to the city, are chiefly taken in the Kurhaus, which contains seventy-five bathing-rooms for mineral water baths, fourteen for peat baths, and two for vapour baths There is another bathing house adjoining the Sprudel colonnade, and another in the temporary *Stadthaus;* they contain twenty-nine bathing-rooms. A new bathing-house for peat baths, which are increasing very much in popularity, has just been commenced, and will be finished in 1880. The peat is taken from the celebrated peat deposits at Franzensbad, where the city of Karlsbad owns a large tract of peat-land.

The following prices are charged for baths :—For a first-class bath(*salon bath*) 1½ florin; for a second-class bath, 1 florin (after 3 o'clock, only ½ florin is charged) ; for a Russian vapour bath, 1 florin ; for a peat bath, 2 to 3 florins, according to the quantity of peat used for it (100 to 200 pounds). Sheets and towels, and warming the bathing-room, are charged extra.

For further information, I also add the *Kurtaxe*, i. e. the fee charged to every visitor for the privilege of drinking as much mineral water as he chooses. Every stranger who remains longer than eight days at Karlsbad must pay this fee, whether he undergoes a bath treatment or not. Visitors are clsssified, as class I., II., III., and IV. Class No. I. comprises the rich ; and as all English, and especially all Americans who visit Europe, are considered rich, they are registered as No. I, and must pay 10 florins *Kurtaxe;* servants and children under fifteen years are charged 1 florin. Physicians and their families pay no tax. Another tax, called *Musik-Taxe*, is imposed for the benefit of the band; it amounts to 5 to 14 florins for each party residing at Karlsbad during the season. There is no exemption from this tax, even physicians being obliged to pay 3 florins for the music.

Karlsbad, though being devoid of the usual *Kurgarten*, with its shady promenades—the pride of almost all German watering places—and the centre of bath life, is surrounded by so many beautiful forests which form one grand park around the city, that the want of a Kurgarten is scarcely felt. There is hardly any watering place on the continent which has such an abundance of shady walks and promenades as Karlsbad has, their entire length having been estimated to be seven German miles (about thirty English miles). They are very well laid out, and gradually lead to the highest points, thereby enabling even feeble persons to ascend the hills without much exertion, and to enjoy the fresh, bracing air. During the warmest days of the season these walks, which are kept in the best order, and liberally provided with a large number of benches, afford pleasant, cool resting-places to invalids.

One of the most delightful promenades of the city is the *Alte Wiese* (old meadow), planted with magnificent old chestnut-trees, and embellished on both sides by shops, exhibiting the latest and handsomest specimens of Bohemian glass ware, garnets, laces, and other articles manufactured in Bohemia. This is the

K

Bazaar of Karlsbad, which is always thronged by a large concourse of strangers, especially in the morning, when they stop there in order to drink the aromatic coffee in front of the celebrated *Café Elephant*, or pass through on the way to the various coffee-gardens outside the city; or in the evening, when they return from concerts and excursions.

Adjoining this promenade is the *Puppsche Allée*, a large square planted with acacia-trees, and adorned with nice flower-beds; on one side is the elegant café, restaurant, and concert-hall of Pupp Brothers, a grand and very well managed establishment; on the other side a handsome spacious colonnade, constructed of iron and glass, belonging to the same proprietors; a pavilion is in the centre of it for the accommodation of the *Kurkapelle*, which plays there twice a week. This square is at present the principal resort of the visitors, especially when the afternoon concerts are advertised.

Leaving this square, we enter the *Kiesweg* (gravel road), a fine promenade, with very old, large trees, and the lively little Tessel on the left side, while the right side is bounded by high hills covered with pine and beech-trees. On this walk we first pass the café and restaurant *Sans-souci*, an elegant building situated on one of the hills, with a fine large garden and a pretty little theatre. About five minutes further up is a bridge, the *Karlsbrücke*. Here the *Kiesweg* ends and the public road commences, with lawns, fields, and hills alternating on both sides. Directly behind the bridge a short promenade leads to two of the most popular coffee-gardens, the one called *Schönbrunn*, the other located on a hill, called *Schweizerhof*. The latter especially is a charming spot, with fresh, pure air. Continuing our promenade along the banks of the river, we pass two other much-favoured coffee-gardens, the *Posthof* and *Trundschaftssaal*, and finally reach the last and most picturesquely situated of all, the *Kaiserpark*, a lovely spot, with handsome flower-beds and fine scenery.

From the large number of coffee-gardens, the reader will surely infer the great importance attributed to resorts of that kind, and this is really the case. Karlsbad's coffee-houses enjoy the reputation of preparing the best coffee ; nowhere else on the continent can you drink such an aromatic coffee with such excellent cream, and nowhere else are you so speedily and cheerfully served as there by the young, active Karlsbad coffee-girls, who promptly execute your orders, eager to earn a *Trinkgeld* (gratuity) of a few kreutzers.

Ascending the hills behind Pupp's restaurant, and turning to the right, we reach, by a short promenade through the woods, the so-called *Hirschensprung* (1520 feet) with a café, and a fine view of the valleys of the Tessel and the Eger. Descending from here, we arrive at the *Fägerhaus*, a little café, once very popular with the guests, but at present chiefly visited by the Karlsbad burghers. Thence by a pleasant promenade of about an hour, gradually ascending, we reach the top of the *Aberg* (1929 feet), one of the highest points in the immediate neighbourhood of Karlsbad. A new coffee-house has lately been erected there. There is also a high tower, from which those who take the trouble of ascending can obtain a fine view of the surrounding country.

Little waggons, drawn by donkeys, carry invalids to all these points for moderate charges.

There are some other interesting points on the hills on the *left* bank of the Tessel, which are very much frequented on account of their pleasant situation, as *Findlater's Tempel*, a wooden structure, erected by Lord Findlater, *Franz-Joseph's Höhe*, where a magnificent high tower, lately erected, affords a fine view, *Freundschaftshöhe*, *Bellevue*, &c., &c.

Just opposite to the Hirschensprung, on the *right* bank of the Tessel, is one of the most popular resorts, on a mountain called the *Drei-Kreuzberg*. We reach it by ascending the hill directly behind the Catholic church; passing through the *Panorama*, a restaurant with a handsome garden and fine view, and crossing the *Prager Strasse*, we enter the woods leading to the top of the mountain, which we reach by half an hour's pleasant walk. On the *Drei-Kreuzberg* (1693 feet) we have a magnificent view. At our feet, in the valley below, we see the city and the surrounding hills; on our right, the charming valley of the Eger, with numerous villages and rich fields; in the background the *Fichtelgebirge*; in the east the *Erzgebirge*. On a plateau, near the top, is a nice little café, and a *camera obscura*, to which you are admitted by paying a fee of ten kreuzers.

There are many other picturesque places in the immediate neighbourhood of the city. Dr. Hlawacek, author of an excellent monograph on Karlsbad (13th edition, 1880, Hans Feller, Karlsbad), enumerates twenty, and more, which can easily be reached on foot, besides fifteen others, easily accessible by carriage. But it would exceed the limits of this treatise to dwell any longer on the description of these places. One, however, must be mentioned, on account of the popularity of its waters; this is GIESS-HÜBEL, a lovely little place, reached by a drive of an hour and a half. It consists of three houses, containing forty rooms for patients. It is very much frequented by excursionists from Karlsbad, has a *Kurhaus*, colonnade, bathing establishment, and fine promenades in the woods. The sale of the mineral water is very large. This water is a very refreshing drink, and is much used in Karlsbad instead of common water.

The inhabitants of Karlsbad are very polite and obliging in their intercourse with the guests, and, like all the inhabitants of all other watering places, they try to make as much money out of the strangers as possible. Living is not cheap, though any one acquainted with the locality, and in the habit of economizing, can live on a comparatively small outlay of money. English and Americans particularly are very welcome, and must be on their guard, especially with regard to hotel-keepers, who usually take advantage of strangers ignorant of the language, laws, and regulations of the place. According to the latter, guests in hotels pay for rooms *by the day*, if they have not made a special arrangement for a longer time, and hotel-keepers have no right to charge for a full week. The best way is to hire a furnished room for the whole term of four or six weeks. The rent is generally paid weekly, some landlords charging an extra fee for service; it is always expedient to settle this point when hiring the room. Servants always expect a gratuity, no matter whether the landlord charges for it on the bill or not. Most of the hotels have furnished rooms to let by the week or month, but in general it is better to live in a private house, there being mostly less noise and more comfort.

The price for furnished rooms varies according to situation and time; from May 15 to July 15 prices are high, afterwards lower. A single room can be had for 5, 10, and 20 florins per week, two or four rooms for 20 to 50 florins, large apartments for 80, 100 and 200 florins per week. Strangers should keep in mind that at every restaurant or *café* they must pay a small gratuity (*Trinkgeld*) to the waiters; even the cashier (*Zahlkellner*), who receives your money, expects something of the kind. Generally a few kreutzers are sufficient. This habit is very disgraceful and annoying, but we are obliged to submit to it.

In regard to the mode of living, diet, exercise, bathing, &c., I refer to the first part of this treatise; all rules laid down in former chapters should be rigidly obeyed by patients undergoing a treatment at the Karlsbad springs. The great reputation and the splendid results attained by these powerful waters are mainly due to the strict observance of the rigid dietetic regimen prescribed and enforced by the bath-physicians.

Entertainments are amply provided for in the shape of the regular daily concerts of the *Kurkapelle*, of extra entertainments given by eminent artists and singers, or by the bands of Hungarian gypsies, or of the regiments of the Austrian army. There are also two theatres, where comedies and operettas are performed, and every Saturday evening a *réunion* takes place at the *Kurhaus* (ladies are requested not to appear in full dress).

A large number of newspapers can also be read at Pupp's *café;* English books can be obtained at the circulating library of Mr. Feller (Alte Wiese).

Hotels: Zum goldenen Schild, Hotel Anger, Stadt Hannover, Paradies, Hôtel de Russie.

Restaurants: Puppe, Salle de Saxe, Kurhaus, San-souci, Loib, &c., &c. There are good restaurants in all hotels.

Physicians: Hochberger, Gans senior, Seegen, Preiss, Anger, Zimmer, Krauss, Meyer, Hoffmann, Neubauer, Hlawacek, London, Schiffer.

Access: From London and Paris, *viâ* Cologne, to Leipzig and Karlsbad, or *viâ* Frankfort on the Main, Bamberg, Eger to Karlsbad; from Bremen or Hamburg, *viâ* Magdeburg, Leipzig to Karlsbad.

By a three hours' railway ride from Karlsbad, we reach

TEPLITZ, with the suburb Schönau, next to Karlsbad the most celebrated and most frequented spa of Austria; situated in a wide, pleasant valley, 700 feet above the sea. It is an old, industrious city, with 14,000 inhabitants, and is one of the oldest watering places of Europe, having celebrated in 1862 its eleventh centenary as a spa. It is a quiet and comparatively cheap place, with splendid gardens, excellent bathing arrangements and beautiful environs. Like Karlsbad, it is visited by invalids from all parts of the globe, the average number of patients being 10,000 annually, who take 280,000 baths. The regular season lasts from the 1st of May until the end of September, but the bathing establishments are open during the whole year, and prices are reduced during the winter. Patients can take baths even on very cold days without any danger of taking cold, as most of the bathing-houses have furnished rooms for the accommodation of bathers, who can retire to their apartments immediately after the bath, thereby avoiding any exposure. There are seven large bathing-houses in Teplitz and two in Schönau, but all are so crowded in the height of the season that patients who neglect to apply for a bathing-room several days before entering on the bath-course have scarcely any chance of getting accommodated at a convenient hour. The arrangements in general are complete; the rooms are large and high, the bathing-tubs of marble or porcelain; to bathe in them is indeed a great luxury.

There is a *Trinkhalle*, where all kinds of bottled mineral waters are sold and drunk. A *Kurgarten*, situated in the centre of the city, is the point of attraction for visitors in the morning from six till eight o'clock, while the band is executing popular compositions of celebrated masters. Here is the *Kursalon* (*Kurhaus*) with two spacious reading-rooms supplied with a large number of English, French, and German newspapers; also the theatre, and the magnificent *Kaiserbad*, with elegantly furnished apart-

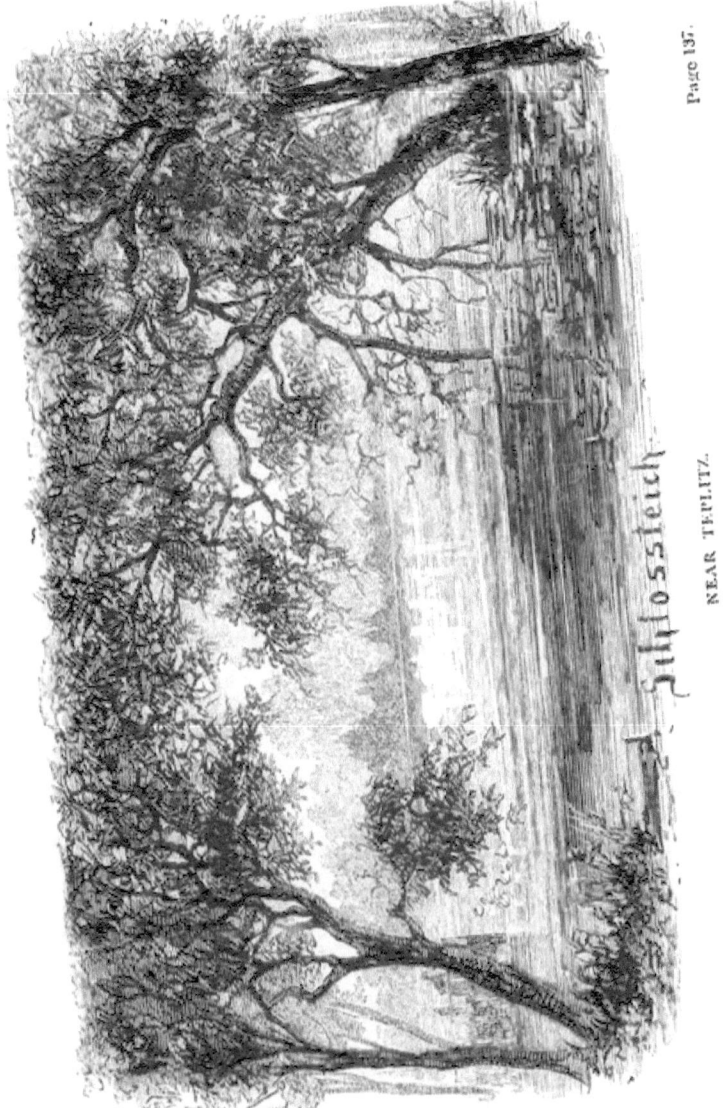

Schlossteich.
NEAR TEPLITZ.

Page 137.

ments and splendid bathing-rooms. From 12 till 1 p.m. the fashionable world crowd in the beautiful park of Prince Clary's Schloss (castle) to listen again to the concert, and to gaze at each other; there is a fine restaurant, where refreshments are served, and *table d'hôte* dinners are prepared.

Several new parks (*Siumepark, Kaiserpark*) and new promenades (*Humbold-, Payer-Anlagen*) have been laid out of late.

Close by the city is the *Königshöhe* (800 feet) and higher up the *Schlackenberg*, a curious structure in the shape of a mediæval castle, built of bricks and slags. A short distance from the city (15 or 25 minutes) are the following interesting points: *Stefanshöhe, Tasanerie, Turnerpark, Bergschlösschen* (1000 feet) and the *Schlossberg*, with the ruins of an old castle razed in 1655. All these points have fine shady promenades and restaurants.

There are also numerous interesting places in the neighbourhood of Teplitz, which can be reached by a few hours' carriage ride. We mention: *Bilin*, reputed for its mineral waters, of which one million bottles are annually exported; *Eichwald*, of late much frequented as a climatic resort for lung diseases; the *Geiersberg*, with old ruins; *Mariaschein*, a noted place of pilgrimage; *Graupen*, an old mountain-city with a celebrated church, and in close proximity the *Wilhelmshöhe* and *Rosenburg; Osegg*, a grand monastery with a large park.

From Teplitz a very interesting excursion is made to the *Milleschauer* or *Donnersberg* (2600 feet), where an unsurpassed fine view is obtained of the largest portion of Bohemia. Visitors take the stage to Pilkau, (two hours), and thence they reach the top of the mountain by an hour's walk.

Finally, I wish to remark that the picturesque *Saxon Switzerland* can easily be reached by railway.

Hotels: Post, König v. Preussen, Stadt London, Schwarzes Ross, Neptun.

Patients are recommended to hire rooms at one of the bathing-houses; all information is readily given by the *Bade-Inspection* (the superintendents of baths) of the city (for English and Americans in the English language).

Restaurants: Kursalon, Gartensalon at Clary's park, Felsenkeller, Drei Rosen, Germania, and at all hotels.

Physicians: Drs. Höring, Richter, Seiche, Willigk, Eberle, Hirsch, Delhaes, Kraus, Karner, Lustig, Heller, Redlich, Rezek, Karnim.

Access: From London or Paris, *viâ* Cologne and Leipzig, or *viâ* Frankfort on the Main and Bamberg to Eger, thence to Teplitz; from Hamburg or Bremen, *viâ* Leipzig and Eger, or *viâ* Dresden and Bodenbach, to Teplitz.

Starting from Karlsbad, and pursuing a south-westerly course, we reach, by a three hours' railway ride, the third of Bohemia's far-famed watering places,

MARIENBAD, a place considerably patronized by the English. It is a little city, with 3000 inhabitants, 1932 feet above the sea, an exceedingly charming spot, situated in an open valley, and surrounded on three sides by high, thickly-wooded hills. The air is moist and pretty cool in the morning and evening.

This place—a hundred years ago an inaccessible wilderness—was in 1818 established as a watering place; Goethe sojourned there in 1820, drinking the powerful waters; everything, however, was so unsettled that he wrote to a friend: "I feel as if I were in the American solitudes, where the forests are cut down in order to build up a city within three years." It is now a superb, rising place, with elegant hotels, neat villas, large lodging-houses, and many pleasant promenades. The arrangements for drinking and bathing are very good; the numerous cafés and restaurants equal those of Karlsbad. But prices are higher than at the other Bohemian spas. The great efficacy of the springs has raised Marienbad to the rank of a *world-spa*, about 9000 patients visiting it during the season; one million bottles of the Marienbad *Kreuzbrunnen* are annually exported to all parts of the world.

This *Kreuzbrunnen*, the most celebrated of the springs, is enclosed by a fine rotunda, with a high cupola, a large gilded cross on the top of the latter attracting the attention of the patients to that important spot; on each side are added pretty colonnades, inclosing a little lawn, where the bust of Dr. Nihr, the founder of Spa Marienbad, has been placed on a pedestal of red Bohemian marble. Adjoining the Kreuzbrunnen is a beautiful shady promenade, 900 feet long, where patients walk about during the two morning hours (6 till 8) which they devote to the goddess of the spring. A long brick building, close to the Kreuzbrunnen, is used for promenading on rainy days, and adjoins another building, containing two rows of shops, the *Bazaar*, where genuine Bohemian goods, as garnets, laces, glass-ware, &c., are sold. The most abundant of all Marienbad springs is the *Ferdinandsbrunnen*, about twenty minutes distant from the spa; its water is carried by pipes to the promenade, where it flows into a vase of alabaster. Another spring, the *Waldquelle*, situated in a pleasant ravine in the woods, about five minutes distant from the Kreuzbrunnen, is the place of rendezvous from half-past eleven to half-past twelve, at which time the band plays. There are six other springs, which are used for drinking or bathing, the most interesting of all being the *Marienquelle*. This spring, immensely rich in carbonic acid, is used only for bathing. A large basin (30 feet by 75, and 6 feet deep), enclosed by a common unsightly building, is filled with the mineral water, which issues from the bottom; there are ten or twelve wells, which break forth with a murmuring sound caused by the innumerable gas bubbles with which the water is impregnated. In the same basin are hundreds of gas-wells, which throw out pure carbonic acid, and keep the surface of the water in perpetual motion. The quantity of the carbonic acid is so great that a space of two feet height above the water is thoroughly impregnated with it, and a burning candle lowered to the surface of the water is immediately extinguished.

Marienbad has a pretty *Kurgarten*, with lawns and bosquets, alternating with pleasant walks. A large building, called *Stadthaus*, in which the post and telegraph-offices are located, contains a *concert-salon* and a reading-room (with the London *Times* and *Daily News*).

Notwithstanding the large number of hotels and lodging-houses, it is often impossible in the height of the season to be accommodated with a room; it is therefore advisable to apply for one in writing several days in advance.

Two large bathing-houses, the *alte* and *neue Badhaus*, contain 130 bathing-rooms for mineral water, peat, iron, and vapour baths; carbonic acid baths are also applied. The peat baths are very popular, as they are considered very efficacious in rheumatic and gouty swellings, tumors of the spleen, &c.

The season begins in May, and lasts until the end of September; in the height of it the spa is crowded by the fashionable society, and bath-life is very lively. Those who enjoy the sight of large, fat persons of immense weight, hardly able to move about, and anxious to rid themselves of their burden, can be fully pleased by going to the Kreuzbrunnen promenade; there they can see them by the hundreds, resignedly swallowing considerable quantities of the salutary spring.

Marienbad is a very convenient place for promenading, the pine-woods being easily accessible from each house, pleasant, shady walks leading gradually up to the top of the hills. One of the nearest and most frequented promenades is the one to the *Cross* on the *Hamelikaberg;* other promenades are—to the *Hirtenruhe, Friedrichstein, Mersery-Tempel, Friedrich-Wilhelmshöhe,* &c. A very popular excursion is one made to the *Podhorn*, a basalt-mountain an hour and a half distant from Marienbad, with pavilions, resting-places and a restaurant.

Hotels: Klinger, Englischer Hof, Stadt Hamburg, Stadt Weimar, Stadt Warschau, Hotel Stern, Bellevue, Neptun.

Coffee-houses : Bellevue, Mühlig, Waldschlucht, Panorama, Jaegerhaus, Ferdinandsmühle, &c., &c.

Restaurants: Kursaal, Bellevue, Delfin, Tepler Haus, Stadt München.

Physicians: Drs. Basch, Herzig, Fränkl, Schneider, Lucca, Kisch, Schindler, Porges, Loewy, Ott, Heidler, &c., &c.

Access: From London or Paris, viâ Frankfort on the Main, Bamburg, Eger to Marienbad ; from Bremen or Hamburg, viâ Leipzig, Reichenbach, Eger to Marienbad.

We shall now visit the fourth and last of the celebrated Bohemian spas, the well-known ladies' bath,

FRANZENSBAD, two hours and a half from Karlsbad (by railway). It is situated 1570 feet above the sea in an open plain, devoid of all attractions ; the air is pure and fresh, but sudden changes of temperature often occur. This spa presents a fine, aristocratic appearance, and consists of 150 houses, all erected for the sole purpose of receiving patients. Most of the visitors are ladies, the iron-springs and the peat baths being considered highly beneficial for quite a number of female complaints. The number of visitors is about 8000 annually, with only a small number of gentlemen. The largest public building is the *Kurhaus*, with a grand *salon*, 115 feet long, 52 feet wide. There are two colonnades, a wooden one at the *Franzensquelle*, extending to the *Kurhaus*, with many shops, and another one, which is a long brick building (221 paces), at the *Salzquelle*, both used for promenading on rainy days. They are surrounded by fine pleasure-grounds. Many elegant hotels and villas, most of them situated in gardens, afford charming but not cheap residences for invalids, living being considered very high at Franzensbad. A large park extending from the city to the railway station affords pleasant and ample opportunity for outdoor exercise.

Nearly the whole colony of patients assemble in the park in the afternoon from 4.30 to 6.30 p.m., when the usual concert takes place. Bath-life here is dull, the majority of the patients being feeble and suffering, and not disposed to indulge in any extravagance. Three large bathing establishments, Dr. Cortellieri's, Mr. Loihmann's, and Stadt Egerer, containing 315 bathing-rooms, can accommodate a very large number of patients; they are excellently arranged and very well managed; 120,000 baths are given during the season, half of them being peat baths. The Franzensbad peat has a greater reputation than any other, owing to the great quantity of sulphate of iron which it contains. A new bathing-house is in the course of erection.

Hotels: Hotel Adler, British Hotel, Hotel Gieseln Holzer, Hübner, Müller, Kreuz, Leipzig, Kaiservilla, Wessel, all with restaurants.

Restaurants : Kursaal, Weilburg, Bahnhof, Brandenburger Thor (with a nice garden), Prince of Wales (with a garden).
Physicians : Drs. Cortellieri, Köstler, Boschau, Kohn, Meissl, Fellner, Sommer, Dissl, &c., &c.
Access : The same as to Marienbad.

By an hour's railway ride from Franzensbad we reach

ELSTER, a comparatively new spa, as it has existed as a watering-place only thirty years, but already very popular. It lies in a wooded, romantic mountain region, 1465 feet above the sea, has 1250 inhabitants, and excellent arrangements. The principal wells are the *Eisenquelle, Moritzquelle,* and *Salzquelle,* all located in a fine *Kurgarten,* and covered by handsome buildings, where the patients promenade when unfavourable weather forbids active exercise in the *Kurgarten ;* there are also good appliances for warming the mineral water for the benefit of patients with whom the cold water does not agree. The large *bathing-house* contains 134 bathing-rooms, twenty-four of which are used for peat-baths; the bathing-tubs are of copper, and on cool days the rooms are heated by steam-coils. A large reading-room is on the second floor of the same building. Elster does not yet enjoy the costly pleasure of a grand *Kurhaus,* but there is a large concert-room called *Kursaal,* in the Hôtel de Saxe, where *réunions* and concerts take place. The spa is surrounded by magnificent forests. The number of visitors already amounts to 5000 annually.

Hotels: Hôtel de Saxe, Bauer, Wittiner Hof.
Physicians: Drs. Flechsig, Löbner, Cramer, Peters, Paessler, Hahn.
Access: The same as to Marienbad.

There is a charming little spa, called—

JOHANNISBAD, in the Bohemian Riesengebirge, near the Silesian frontier; though a little out of the usual route of tourists, it deserves to be noticed on account of its picturesque situation, and the curative action of its thermal waters. It is a rising spa, which in 1859 had only 200 visitors, but in 1875 already over 2000. It is a little village of seventy houses, situated 1955 feet above the sea, in a narrow, wooded valley. It has a pure, bracing forest-and-mountain air, rich in ozone, and is considered an excellent climatic resort for persons who feel debilitated after having completed a severe course of treatment at Karlsbad or Marienbad. There are two large basins for common baths, and bathing-rooms for single baths. Fresh wheys are prepared every day. There is a handsome wooden colonnade, 140 feet long, and 20 feet wide, for promenading and concerts; also a *Kursaalhaus*, with a fine *salon* and reading-room.

The cool, balsamic pine-forests in the immediate neighbourhood afford very pleasant resting-places and walks on warm summer days. Concerts are given twice a week in the *forest-park*.

A number of interesting places are suitable points for excursions; of these I mention the *Ladig*, a mountain south of Johannisbad, with a restaurant, and a grand view; the *Klausengraber*, a narrow, steep,

L

romantic defile; the *Hoffmannsbande* (2468 feet). Those able to make longer excursions may visit the *Schneekoppe* (5066 feet), the highest mountain in Northern Germany, the *Hübnerbande* (3200 feet), &c., &c.

Hotels: Kurhaus, Preussicher Hof, Kaiser von Oesterreich, Villa Bohemia, Kronprinz Rudolf, Stadt Prag, Deutsches Haus.

Physicians: Drs. Kopf, Pauer, Schreyer.

Access: From Dresden or Berlin, viâ Görlitz to station Freiheit, thence by a half-hour's stage drive to Johannisbad.

2. THE SPAS IN UPPER AND LOWER AUSTRIA AND SALZBURG.

In order to visit these spas we start from *Vienna*, the magnificent capital of the Austrian Empire, the most pleasant of the large continental cities, and a great favourite with strangers, owing to the civility of its inhabitants, the good living, and the beautiful environs.

By a short railway ride we reach the celebrated sulphur spa—

BADEN, the favourite summer residence of the well-to-do Vienna citizens, very much frequented by invalids and tourists, on account of the delightful situation, good arrangements, and charming surroundings. It is a fine little city, with 7500 inhabitants, situated 672 feet above the sea, on the slope of the *Wiener Wald*. The air, a mountain air, is pure and bracing, but subject to sudden changes of temperature. There are thirteen springs, which were already used by the Romans. A dark, close passage-way, ninety feet long, leads to the principal well, called *Römerquelle;* those who are not afraid of a little perspiration may pass through it, and will find at the end the hot spring breaking forth in a big stream from a depth of eighteen feet. Some patients enter it for the purpose of inhaling the hot vapours—a very undesirable practice, the place being too uncomfortable. Baden has fifteen bathing establishments, with society baths, and single bathing-rooms, the former being the most popular; one of these establishments, the *Herzogsbad*, can accommodate 150 bathers. The common, or society baths, where ladies and gentlemen bathe together, have galleries accessible to visitors who wish to converse with the bathers, or to take a look at the proceedings. Of course all bathers are dressed in long bathing-gowns; and I am bound to say that the utmost decency prevails, the rules and regulations being very strict. The attendants are very obliging, and well trained. Bathers, on emerging from the water, are very carefully rubbed off with warm towels and sheets. Baden has also a grand *swimming-bath* (160 feet by 40 feet), filled with thermal water of 76°. The spa has a fine, shady Kurgarten, a nice Trinkhalle, and a large number of beautiful promenades; of these, I particularly recommend the walk to the *Helenenthal*. The number of guests is about 10,000 annually.

Ten minutes distant from Baden by railway is the little spa—

VÖSLAU, a lovely little spot, with an immense swimming-bath, filled with thermal water of 77°. The bath, which is delightfully situated in the woods, has a very large number of dressing-rooms, and strong douches and shower-baths. There is also a smaller swimming-bath for ladies. Good restaurant and nice promenades are in the immediate vicinity. Vöslau is an excellent place for a summer resort, and as such can be recommended to foreigners residing at Vienna.

Hotels at Baden: Stadt Wien, Hotel Munsch, Schwarze Adler, Hirsch, Löwe.

Physicians: Drs. Landesmann, Roller, Mülleitner.

Travelling from Vienna, either by steamboat up the Danube, or by railway, we arrive at Linz, a city worth visiting, owing to its fine situation. From here, by a two hours' railway ride, we arrive at Steyer, thence by a two hours' stage ride, we reach

HALL, a place of repute, on account of the iodine and bromine springs. It is charmingly situated in a romantic Alpine region, 1064 feet above the sea; the climate is mild, and moderately moist. Hall is a pretty town, with 1000 inhabitants, and a large number of hotels and lodging-houses. It has a handsome *Kurhaus*, with a fine concert *salon*, a billiard and reading-room, with a large number of newspapers. (No English newspapers). The lower story of this building is occupied by the baths, there being eighty-five bathing-rooms, with tubs of cement, porcelain, or marble. The last named are very elegant indeed.

An extensive *Kurpark*, with fine shady walks, adjoins the *Kurhaus*. A long brick building, a short distance from the Kurhaus, called *Wandelbahn*, is used for promenading on rainy days. Patients there drink the water of the celebrated *Thassiloquelle*, which for 1100 years has enjoyed a great reputation in scrofulous affections. The water has a refreshing, but very salty taste. The spring issues from the earth, several hundred feet distant, in the valley below; but for the convenience of the invalids, the mineral water is carried to the fountain in the Wandelbahn by means of a force-pump. On the whole, the place seems very quiet, the only noise noticed there being made by the music-band, which plays several times a day, whether it be for the enjoyment or the torture of the unfortunate patients, is hard to say. About 2000 patients annually visit this charming spa, scrofulous children contributing a large portion of the patronizers.

Hotels: Kaiserin Elisabeth is the largest hotel, with high prices. There are numerous other hotels and lodging-houses.

Physicians: Loewy, Kaster, Pachner, Rabl, Schuber.

Access: From London, *viâ* Frankfort, Regensburg, Linz, to Steyer; from Paris, *viâ* Strasburg, München, Linz, to Steyer; from Bremen or Hamburg, *viâ* Leipzig, Regensburg, Linz, to Steyer; thence by stage to Hall.

By a three and half hours' railway ride from Linz we reach—

ISCHL, *the gem of the Austrian spas.* There is hardly a lovelier and more idyllic spot to be found on the continent than this charming little place, which is surrounded by a large number of beautiful Alpine lakes, and by high, picturesque mountains of 5000 feet elevation. It is situated 1530 feet above the sea, and is the centre of the far-famed *Salzkammergut*, an Alpine region, hardly surpassed anywhere in beauty of scenery. The climate is equally moist and mild, very suitable for persons suffering with affections of the lungs. Its romantic scenery and salubrious climate have already rendered Ischl one of the most frequented and fashionable spas of Austria, it being especially patronized by the Emperor Francis Joseph, the Austrian nobility, and the monied aristocracy of Vienna. Number of inhabitants, 4000.

In the height of the season it is crowded to the utmost; rooms are extremely scarce, and prices very high. There is a good deal of elegance, but no extravagance at this spa. The bathing arrangements are excellent, the bathing-rooms being commodious and airy; the tubs are excavations in the floor, and are lined with granite. Near the bath-house is a large, one-story building, where mineral waters and whey are served, and where the band plays in the morning when the weather is unfavourable. Of all the Austrian spas, Ischl has the handsomest *Kurhaus* (*casino*), with large and elegant *salons*, restaurant, and reading-room, and a grand terrace, where the visitors take coffee or other refreshments while listening to the concert. A fine garden, shady walks, and promenades surround the *Kurhaus*. The principal promenade, called the *Esplanade*, is on the left bank of the little river Traun; it is a fine shady walk, with linden and acacia-trees, the centre of attraction in the evening, when the band plays. There are many interesting points to which the visitors promenade, as: the *Sophien-Doppelblick*, with a grand view of the snow-covered *Dachstein; Kalvarienberg, Karolinen-Panorama, Hundskogel*, &c. The imperial villa and park are open to the public when the Emperor is absent. All the surroundings are beautiful. Elegant villas, built on prominent points, are great ornaments to the place.

Very interesting excursions are made to Hallstadt, Gosau, to the Schafberg, Salzburg, &c.

Hotels: Kaiserin Elisabeth, Hotel Baur, Post, Kreuz, Stern, Erzherzay Karl, Krone.

Physicians: Drs. Heinemann, Fürstenburg, Hertzka, Hirschfeld, Kaan, Pfost, Stieger, Scheiring, Schütz.

Access: From Linz, by railway to Ischl; or from Linz to Gmunden by railway; thence by steamboat over the *Traunsee* to Ebensee, thence by railway to Ischl—a very interesting trip.

From Ischl the railway takes us in an hour and a half to the little spa—

AUSSEE, a small place, with 1400 inhabitants; situated 2100 feet above the sea, in a beautiful Alpine region (although situated in Styria, I mention it here on account of its proximity to Ischl). It is very well sheltered from rough winds by the surrounding hills and mountains. Since a few years Aussee has come into great popularity, and already enjoys the patronage of 2800 visitors annually; as a natural consequence it has been endowed with a plain little building styled *Kurhaus*, and high prices. Its brine

(*Saale*) is stronger than that of any other saline spa. Aussee is eminently suitable for a climatic health-resort, owing to its high and pleasant situation and pure mountain air.

Excursions to Altaussee, Grundelsee, Hallstadt, are highly recommended.

Hotels: Flackel, Post, Sonne.

Physicians: Drs. Schreiber, Pohl.

Access: The same as to Ischl.

From Aussee we continue our railway travel through the pleasant valleys of the Enno and Salzach to Lend, a station on the Salzburg-Wörgl railway, and thence by stage to—

GASTEIN. The trip from Lend to Gastein is very interesting, the whole region being picturesque in the highest degree. A narrow road leads up the hills. On one side it is bounded by steep rocks, while on the other, in a deep ravine, the water of the wild mountain rivulet, *Ache*, pursues its boisterous course. After passing through a narrow, gloomy defile, called *Klamm Pass*, we enter the pleasant, romantic Gastein valley. We soon reach *Hof-Gastein*, a small town with 800 inhabitants, 2800 feet above the sea. Many invalids stop here, as the rooms are cheaper than at *Bad Gastein*, the thermal waters are carried down from the spa by pipes, the temperature thereby being lowered a few degrees. After a further drive of one hour, always ascending, on a very good waggon-road, we arrive at the celebrated spa *Wildbad Gastein*, 3400 feet above the sea. It has the highest elevation of all so-called indifferent thermal spas of central

Europe. It is situated at the foot of the *Graukagl*, (7667 feet), and on the left bank of the *Ache*, which, in the immediate vicinity, precipitates itself from the steep rocks with a thundering noise, forming two magnificent waterfalls. The whole scenery is grand and picturesque. For want of space, one house was built somewhat above the other, so that at a distance they look as if fastened to the side of the steep mountain.

The climate is Alpine, with a fresh, invigorating air; however, sudden and frequent changes of temperature sometimes occur, and even during the season, in July and August, there are many cool and rainy days. Patients are therefore earnestly reminded to provide themselves with warm clothing. Prices are high, and rooms always very scarce; the little spa is annually visited by more than 3000 persons, and is very crowded during July and August. Patients desirous of living at the Wildbad, should send orders for rooms some time before their intended arrival. Gastein has gained great reputation through Emperor William of Germany, who has patronized the spa for many years. The higher and more refined classes of society are well represented. To be sure, there is no luxurious bath-life at the little watering place, no excitement and no extravagance; everything goes on quietly and pleasantly, all the visitors being really sick, and desirous of being restored to health.

The bathing arrangements are perfect; the bathing-rooms are large, airy, and elegant. The thermal water is perfectly pure and clear, without any deposit; bathers experience a delightful feeling of ease while remaining in it, and feel highly refreshed and enlivened after having finished the bath. The usual inevitable *Kurhaus* is not at Gastein ; instead of it there is a long, wooden structure, with a great many glass windows, which afford a magnificent view of the valley ; on rainy days patients promenade here. I have also noticed some newspapers in this building. However, there are a good many fine walks near the spa, and some opportunity is offered for pleasant and interesting excursions. We mention especially, the one to the *Stassfeld*, a lovely green plateau, surrounded by a grand mountain scenery.

Hotels : 1, in Hof Gastein : Moser, Gruber, Kreuz, Meisset ; 2, in Wildbad Gastein : Straubinger, Hirsch, Grabenwirth, Hotel Badeschloss.

Physicians : in Hof Gastein : Dr. Pfeiffer ; in Wildbad : Drs. Bunzel, Haerdtl, Pröll, Schider, Hoenigsberg.

Access : From London or Paris, to Munich, thence *viâ* Salzburg to station Lend, thence by stage to Gastein ; from Bremen or Hamburg, to Munich, Salzburg, Lend, &c.

3. THE SPAS IN THE SOUTHERN PART OF AUSTRIA.

These baths, with the exception of the little spa *Villach*, are situated in Styria. They are not so well known to English and Americans as they deserve to be on account of their pleasant situation and the efficacy of their thermal waters. At present they are mainly patronized by the better classes of Austrian society. Accommodations are everywhere good, and charges for board, baths, &c., moderate ; at some places even low. As there is no display, no high bath-life at these watering places, they are eminently fitted for invalids who desire a cheap, comfortable resort, and refined society.

We commence our trip by travelling from Vienna, on the Austrian Southern railway, to Gratz, passing the celebrated *Semmering Pass*. *Gratz*, the capital of Styria, is most picturesquely situated on both banks of the river Mur; it has a fine promenade and a celebrated view on the *Schlossberg*, (1500 feet), the popular resort of the good citizens of Gratz, and of the many strangers who permanently reside there on account of the beautiful situation and the cheapness of living. There are two watering places in the neighbourhood of Gratz, Tobelbad and Gleichenberg.

GLEICHENBERG is very picturesquely situated, in a narrow, fertile valley, 900 feet above the sea, protected by mountains against north and west winds, sheltered from the east by wooded hills, and open only to the south. The climate is mild, and very steady, without any sudden changes, the air pure and moderately moist. The houses are very pleasantly situated in a large park. Owing to the excellent climate and efficacious springs, the spa has become a favourite resort for patients afflicted with lung diseases. Milk and whey cures are much *en vogue* here; there is also a room for the inhalation of pine-needle extract. About 4000 persons visit the place annually. There are five springs, the *Constantinquelle* being the most popular. Two others, the *Klausen* and *Johannisbrunnen*, about an hour distant from Gleichenberg, contain iron, and are much used.

Hotels: Stadt Mailand, Stadt Venedig, Stadt Würzburg, Vereinshaus, Villa Höflingen.
Physicians: Drs. Hausen, Klar, Weiss, Netwald, Zavori, Rowitz.
Access: From Vienna, *viâ* Gratz to station Fildbach, thence by an hour's stage ride to Gleichenberg.

TOBELBAD is a pretty little place in the immediate neighbourhood of Gratz, 1070 feet above the sea, in a narrow, pleasant valley, surrounded by pine-woods; many villas are pleasantly situated on the slopes of the shady hills. Everything looks neat and very well arranged. There are two large common or society baths, and twenty single bathing-rooms. The charges for lodgings, baths, servants, and even for boot-blacking, are fixed by the administration of the spa, and are very moderate indeed. There is a nice little *Kurhaus*, and a handsome wooden structure in semi-circular shape (180 feet long), for concerts and for promenading on rainy days. A nice garden is laid out in front of the *Kurhaus;* a number of shady walks in the surrounding pine forests afford pleasant opportunity for out-door exercise. The number of patients is small (about 600 annually), but many tourists, and citizens of Gratz, visit the place.

Hotels: There are about nine buildings, under the special supervision of the bath director, where furnished rooms can be hired for one florin a day, and less; besides these, rooms can be hired in many private houses.

Physician: Dr. Blumauer.
Access: From Gratz, by half an hour's railway ride

to station Premstten, thence by a fine promenade through the pine forest in twenty minutes to Tobelbad.

Travelling south from Gratz, by railway, we reach in two and a half hours the small station Pöltschach, and thence by stage we arrive at—

ROHITSCH, more celebrated, and far more popular, than the preceding spa. It is situated 750 feet above the sea, in a beautiful valley, sheltered from the north by wooded mountains, while the south wind has free access; the climate therefore is very mild. The arrangements are good, and the prices moderate. This spa, together with Tobelbad and Neuhaus, belongs to the province of Styria, and the prices of all requisites are fixed by the provincial government. The government buildings are provided with sixty bathing-rooms, and 341 furnished rooms for patients. The surroundings are beautiful, and afford ample opportunity for excursions (to the Donatiberg, 2800 feet high, &c.) About 3000 patients annually patronize the place, and 2,000,000 bottles of the water are exported every year.

Physicians: Drs. Sock, Fröhlich, Schüler.

The next station to Pöltschach on the Austrian Southern railway is *Cilli*, a handsome old city, founded by the Roman Emperor Claudius. By a very pleasant drive of an hour and a half, either by diligence or carriage, we reach another spa—

NEUHAUS, 1200 feet above the sea, in a charming valley, surrounded on three sides by mountains of

3000—4000 feet elevation. It is the highest of all Styrian baths; nevertheless, the climate is mild and temperate, with a pure mountain air; owing to the abundance of pine forests the air is rich in ozone. The large *Kurhaus* and other establishments are situated in the centre of a fine park; a large *salon* in the *Kurhaus* is supplied with a number of newspapers; twice a day the band gives concerts.

There are two large common baths and several single bathing-rooms, all very well arranged, with good attendance. Patients after arriving are obliged to take their first bath in so-called *Fremdenbad* (stranger's bath) and only after this proceeding are they admitted to the common bath used by the other patients. I consider this rule, which at this spa is strictly observed, a very good one for watering places where common baths are in practice; but I must confess that Neuhaus is the only place where I have found such a rule established and carried out. There are 200 furnished rooms in the lodging-houses for the accommodation of invalids, all under the administration of the provincial government. Charges for board and baths are very moderate.

The environs being very pleasant, ample opportunity is offered for active exercise and excursions. Number of visitors, about 1000.

Physician: Dr. Paltauf.

Access: From Vienna, by railway to Cilli, thence by stage.

Half an hour from Cilli, on the same railway, is—
TÜFFER, with the new bath, *Franz-Joseph's Bad*.

It is situated on the left bank of the river Sann, 690 feet above the sea, and is a pleasant, modest-looking place. The handsome *Kurhaus* is very pleasantly situated in the centre of a shady *Kurgarten*, and has a fine *salon* for concerts, a dining and reading-room, with a few newspapers. The bathing arrangements are very good; there is a fine large common bath, and quite a number of single bathing-rooms, all supplied by three wells, which furnish an abundance of thermal water of 100°. Prices are moderate.

Hotels: There are 152 rooms in the Kurhaus and the adjoining buildings. The following hotels are in the village a short distance from the bath: Brauhaus Villa Stein, &c.

Physician: Dr. Henn.

Access: Directly from Vienna, *viâ* Gratz to station Tüffer.

Far more elegant than Tüffer is—

RÖMERBAD, fifteen minutes from Tüffer by railway, delightfully located on a high hill, in the centre of a fine garden, 730 feet above the sea. This spa appears to be the most fashionable of the Styrian thermal baths; the bathing arrangements are excellent, especially those of the twelve single bathing-rooms. There is also a very large common bath. Prices are higher than at the other Styrian baths. There are very fine pleasure-grounds in the surroundings. The establishment contains 304 rooms for the accommodation of visitors. Number of patients, 1000 annually.

Physicians: Drs. Bunzel, Mayrhofer.

Access: From Vienna, *viâ* Gratz to station Römerbad.

By a beautiful railway ride of seven hours through one of the finest portions of Styria and Carinthia, we arrive at *Killach*, a very old city, 1500 feet above the sea, very picturesquely situated in a wide valley. Half an hour distant from the city, at the foot of the Dobratsch (7000 feet) lies a little spa—

Warmbad VILLACH, to which I desire to direct the attention of English and American tourists and patients. It is a lovely little spot, very secluded, and out of the general route of travellers, but for that very reason a suitable resort for persons desiring rest and comfort. The bathing arrangements are plain but good. I especially mention the large common baths, with a delightful, clear thermal water of 86°, which constantly issues from the sandy grouud. The pretty little *Kurhaus*, with a fine garden, is in close proximity to the railway station. Extensive pine forests adjoin the *Kurhaus*, and afford a pleasant, cool resort on warm days. On the whole, the little spa, though only a very short time in existence, already makes a very fine impression on the visitor.

Lodgings can be had at the Kurhaus, or in the city of Villach: Hotel Tarmann.

A few words may be added on some of the Tyrolese watering places. There are a great many in the picturesque *Pusterthal*, which of late has become very popular with tourists. These spas, however, though highly praised in some guide-books, cannot be recommended to English or Americans. The bathing arrangements being mostly too primitive, and devoid of all and every comfort. The most renowned is the little sulphur spa—

INNICHEN, half an hour distant from the railway station Innichen, 4165 feet above the sea, beautifully situated in a pine forest. Notwithstanding the high elevation, the climate is not rough, the place being sheltered against rough winds by high wooded hills. The air is a fresh, invigorating mountain air. There is no great virtue in the mineral water, and the bathing arrangements are very plain. However, the place is an excellent health resort, and as such it deserves the highest praise, and can be recommended to all patients who are in need of pure, bracing mountain air. There are fifty rooms for the accommodation of patients. Prices for board are very moderate. The rooms are plain and clean, and scarce in the height of the season. The table is good and substantial, although not for *gourmands*. The social intercourse is very pleasant.

Physician, and proprietor : Dr. Scheiber.

Access : From Munich, *viâ* Innsbruck and Franzensfeste to station Innichen, thence by carriage in thirty minutes to the bath.

CHAPTER III.

THE WATERING PLACES OF SWITZERLAND.

SWITZERLAND, the promised land of all tourists, has a considerable number of watering places, most of which have been endowed by nature with very efficacious springs, and with that salubrious fresh mountain air which induces so many thousands to resort to the Swiss Alpine regions. There are so many Englishmen and Americans who make a tour through Switzerland, that a knowledge of the most frequented and most efficacious springs will be useful to them, in case they should desire to stop at a watering place.

I shall only mention the most important of the Swiss spas, adding the names of a few which deserve a passing notice, for the benefit of those who prefer a quiet, secluded place.

Entering Switzerland at Basle, we arrive, after a two hours' railway ride, at the celebrated spa—

BADEN, a place already very well known to the Romans, who called it *Aquæ Helveticæ*. During the middle ages it was the most popular watering place in Europe, and was visited by many thousand guests, from all countries and of all classes of society, especially by many priests, monks, and nuns. It was the place where, in those good old times, the greatest immorality prevailed. It was the fashionable spa, with all kinds of amusements and dissipations. To-day it is chiefly visited by Swiss people and Frenchmen, numbering from 12,000 to 14,000 annually.

It is situated in the valley of the Limmat, 1200 feet above the sea. The larger and more elegant establishments are located on the left bank of the river, while the smaller bathing-houses are on the right bank, and are chiefly visited by the neighbouring countrypeople. There is no fashionable bath life at Baden, the place is quiet and dull. Patients go thither for the purpose of being cured, not for the sake of amusement.

The most complete establishment at Baden is the *Neue Kuranstalt Baden*, with 152 furnished rooms in the main building for the accommodation of invalids, and a large number of furnished rooms in adjoining buildings, called *independances*. The establishment has elegant *salons*, and a reading-room with some English papers (*Galignani's Messenger, Swiss Times*). A moderate number of English and Americans patronize the place. There are over one hundred bathing-rooms in the lower part of the building ; the tubs are excavations in the floor, lined with marble. Cold and warm douches are frequently and skilfully applied by the *doucheurs* and *frotteurs;* also sitz-baths, with very practical appliances for ascending and circular douches.

Baden has a handsome *Kurhaus*, with a fine concert *salon*, an elegant dining-room, a billiard and reading-room, and a small *Kurgarten*, where shady walks are yet a *desideratum*.

Hotels: Kuranstalt Baden, Schiff, Limmathof, Schweizerhof, Freihof, &c.

Physicians: Drs. Diebold, Minnich, Schmitz, Schneubeli, Hephaus, Wagener.

Access: From London, *viâ* Frankfort; from Paris, *viâ* Strasburg; from Bremen or Hamburg, *viâ* Cassel and Frankfort, to Basle and Baden.

From Baden we travel by railway *viâ* Zürich, passing the beautiful Zürich and Wallen lakes, to station Ragatz, a route very much favoured by tourists visiting Chur and the famous *Via Mala*. We leave the railway at Ragatz to visit—

RAGATZ-PFÄFFERS, an old spa, of great, well-merited reputation, acquired by its efficacious thermal waters, and the fresh, pure Alpine air. Ragatz, 1690 feet above the sea, is a charming open village, with 1800 inhabitants, and much visited by tourists, of whom about 50,000 pass through it annually on their way to the far-famed *Tamina* ravine at Pfäffers. The thermal waters issue at the latter place, and are carried to RAGATZ by means of pipes 13,000 feet long. The climate is mild and equable. This spa is frequented by many patients from all parts of Europe. Prices are moderate.

Switzerland has the reputation of being very expensive, and I find it therefore opportune to remark, that those who know *how* to travel, can live comparatively cheaply here as well as anywhere else. Of course, first-class hotels, especially those exclusively patronized by English and Americans, charge high prices, for which, however, they afford first-class accommodations and excellent board. But there are many excellent hotels and *pensions* (boarding-houses) everywhere in Switzerland, where good board and lodging can be obtained for moderate prices (five and seven francs a day, according to the season). There is no doubt that strangers, especially English and Americans, are sometimes overcharged, but very often it is their own fault. Accustomed to the great comfort of their homes, they become exceedingly troublesome to hotel-keepers, by ordering a great many things with which continental hotels are not always provided, and for which high extra charges are made.

The bathing arrangements in Ragatz are very good. In one of the establishments is a large swimming-bath. There is also a fine *Kurgarten*, reading and billiard-room, &c.

Hotels: Quellenhof and Hof Ragatz, Tammino-Hotel, Schweizerhof, Krone.

Physicians: Drs. Dormann, Jäger, Kaiser.

Access: From Hamburg or Bremen, *viâ* Cassel, Frankfort, Basle, and Zurich, to station Ragatz; from London, *viâ* Frankfort, or *viâ* Paris, Strasburg, Basle.

On a good road, we gradually walk up to the original old thermal springs at PFÄFFERS. This road, along the wild, boisterous Tamina river, bounded on one side by high rocks of 500 to 700 feet elevation, is one of the most romantic and most frequented Alpine roads. After an hour's promenade, we reach the spa—

PFÄFFERS, situated 2130 feet above the sea, at the foot of the Calanda (6500 feet), in a ravine between very high lime rocks. It is a cool place, but not very agreeable to those who feel animated by the warm rays of the sun, which here only shines between 10 a.m. and 4 p.m. But the scenery is sublime, the Tamina ravine being unsurpassed by any other in this country in wild grandeur. In order to get a full view of the grand spectacle we pass through the bathing establishment; having bought an admission ticket (1 franc), we pass through the ravine on a safe, commodious plank road, 2100 feet long—in the depth below, the wild, roaring Tamina; above us, the dark high rocks, which scarcely allow the sun's rays to creep into this gloomy passage, and to diffuse a dim, dusky light. At the end of this passage we enter a long shaft, where the hot springs break forth.

The bathing-house is a very extensive, rather gloomy-looking building, with long corridors, and a very large number of furnished rooms, bathing, dining-rooms, &c., all very plain, with moderate prices; there are large common baths, and single bathing-rooms. The customers recruit chiefly from the poorer native population.

We continue our trip by railway from Ragatz to Chur, and here we take the Swiss diligence to the Engadine—an excellent conveyance; hardly anywhere else is the postal service for the transportation of passengers so well regulated and so well managed as in Switzerland. The most picturesque route from Chur to the Engadine is that over the Albula pass. On this road we pass the little sulphur spa—

ALVENEU, situated 3100 feet above the sea, in a pleasant valley, surrounded by forests; it is a quiet, charming place, and has a new, good bathing establishment (erected 1866). The climate is an Alpine one, with fresh, bracing air and frequent changes of temperature.

The road leads up to an elevation of 7500 feet, presenting everywhere a wild, romantic scenery. Passing through Ponte and Samaden, we reach—

ST. MORITZ, a celebrated iron spa, so highly popular with the English and Americans that it rather looks like an English colony. It is a little village, with 400 inhabitants, and is situated about 6000 feet above the sea. No other iron spa can boast of such a high situation and such a strong, invigorating mountain air. The spa lies in an open low meadow, 280 feet lower than the village. The iron water is rich in carbonic acid, and has a great reputation since olden times. The mean temperature of the place is 53° in July, and 50° in August; sudden changes of temperature often occur. Patients should not neglect to provide themselves with warm clothing, it being rather cool in the latter part of August. Close to the spring is a large, commodious *Kurhaus*, containing *salons*, reading and billiard-rooms, forty-four bathing-rooms, and lodgings for 250 persons. The bathing-rooms do not look very elegant, and the small wooden tubs are surely not very comfortable for bathers. Prices are high, and there is not much of that gay, jovial bath life which renders a sojourn at the German spas so pleasant. But the situation of the place is delightful, and the scenery of the whole region is grand.

There are fine promenades in the woods, and pleasant excursions can be made to *Silvaplana*, *Samaden, Pontresina*, and the grand glaciers of the Bernina chain, and to the *Piz Languard*.

Hotels: Kurhaus, Hotel Victoria, Hôtel du Lac, Hotel Kulm. If St. Moritz is crowded, patients will find lodgings at Samaden, Pontresina and Silvaplana, all these places being in the immediate neighbourgood.

Physicians: Drs. Berry, Biermann, Brügge.

One of the most interesting trips is made from St. Moritz to Pontresina and the Bernina pass (7500 feet), on an excellent road, which affords a magnificent view of the whole Bernina mountain-range and the grand glaciers. South of the pass, at an elevation of 3100 feet, we arrive at—

LE PRESE, a little sulphur spa, delightfully situated at the northern end of the charming little lake of Poschiavo. This little spot is really idyllic, and eminently suitable for persons desirous of remaining a short while at a very quiet and retired place. The climate is very mild, the place being well protected against north and north-east winds. Not far from the lake is a fine *Kurhaus* with a garden; the bathing arrangements are good, there being fifteen bathing-tubs of Italian marble; prices are moderate.

Access: From Chur, by diligence to Le Prese, crossing the Albula or Julier Pass.

A further ride on the Bernina road takes us to

Tiruno, an old city already on Italian territory, and thence to Bormio.

BORMIO is a very old spa, and was extensively patronized by the old Romans. It is near the Swiss frontier, and easily accessible by the Swiss diligence. We consider it proper to turn the attention of English and Americans to this watering place on account of its beautiful situation, pure air, good arrangements, and efficacious thermal waters.

The old city of Bormio lies in the wide green valley of the Adda, 3900 feet above the sea. There is a new and an old bathing establishment; the new bath is half an hour distant from the city and 355 feet higher, while the old original bath is still 300 feet higher than the new one. The old bath was erected by the Romans, and some of their old buildings are still in existence; this bath is almost exclusively used by the country people, the charges being considerably lower than at the new bath. Besides mineral water baths, sulphur mud baths are given. These old buildings are very picturesquely situated on high rocks; near by is the place where the thermal springs issue from the rocks; they furnish an abundance of water of 102°, which is carried down by means of pipes to the new establishment.

This new bathing-house was erected several years ago by a Swiss company. It is a grand building, elegant and comfortable in every respect, with a large number of nicely furnished, neat and clean rooms, large *salons*, dining-rooms, &c. There are sufficient accommodations for 150 to 200 guests. The bathing-rooms are high and airy, the tubs lined with marble and porcelain. A nice pleasure-ground is laid out before the establishment, and good walks lead up the hills. In July and August the place is very much patronized. During the summer the climate is very pleasant, the mild Alpine air being invigorating and exhilarating. The surrounding hills afford a grand view of the valley and the high snow-covered mountains, *Piz Colombano* (9800 feet), *Cima di Piazza* (11,500 feet), *Piz Tresoro*, &c. Ample opportunity is afforded for pleasant excursions to several mountain valleys; a trip to the *Stelvio Pass* (8900 feet), the highest of all the Alpine passes, is exceedingly interesting, the scenery on the whole route being the grandest and most picturesque, hardly surpassed by any other in the Alpine regions.

Physicians: Drs. Bruni, Marturano.

Starting from St. Moritz on a trip to the valley of the boisterous Inn, we reach, after a six hours' drive,—

TARASP, in the Lower Engadine, a renowned watering place, 3800 feet above the sea. The climate is milder than that of St. Moritz, the valley being well sheltered from the north winds by the mountains. The mean temperature in July and August is 52° to 58°. There is a fine park, and a magnificent *Kurhaus*, with splendid *salons*, many furnished rooms for guests, and fifty-six bathing-rooms. More than twenty wells furnish an abundance of a very efficacious alkaline saline water, which is mainly used for drinking. The surroundings are grand; and in conjunction with the powerful springs and excellent arrangements would attract a larger number of patients, if the place were more accessible. Patients who do not wish to live at the *Kurhaus*, will find rooms at *Vulpesa*, which is situated 300 feet higher than Tarasp, at a distance of only one quarter of an hour, an excellent road leading up to it from Tarasp.

Hotels at Vulpesa: Bellevue, Alpenrose, Tell, Steiner. Patients can also be accommodated at *Schuls*, twenty minutes from Tarasp; the hotels at these places have lower rates than the *Kurhaus Tarasp* Several stages carry the patients to the springs in the morning.

Hotels at Schuls: Belvedere, Post, Könz, Helvetia.

Physicians: Drs. Arquint, Killias, Pernisch.

Access: From London, Paris, Bremen, or Hamburg, to Ragatz and Landquart by railway; from the railway station Landquart, the Swiss diligences make the trip to Tarasp in fourteen hours, crossing the Fluela Pass.

A few words remain to be said of a watering place which is unique among the spas, owing to the peculiar mode of treatment which is in practice there. This is—

BAD LEUK, a little village in the canton Wallis, with 660 inhabitants. It is situated 4356 feet above the sea, in a narrow, long mountain valley, in the midst of a sublime Alpine scenery, surrounded by majestic mountains, whose peaks are permanently covered with snow. The climate is rather rough, and frequent changes of temperature occur. The season lasts from May until the end of September, the largest number of visitors being there in July and August. Swiss and French chiefly patronize the spa.

There are five great bathing establishments, containing fourteen large common or society baths. In these, invalids of both sexes bathe together, dressed in long bathing-gowns, drinking coffee, chatting, reading, or playing cards or chess on little tables floating on the water. There are separate dressing-rooms, and separate entrances to the baths for each sex. In the bathing-rooms galleries are erected for lookers-on or friends of the bathers who wish to converse with them There are twenty-two springs, which furnish such an immense quantity of thermal water of 92° to 122° that nine-tenths of it flows into the river Dala, being entirely superfluous. The treatment is very peculiar and old-fashioned; bathers remain in the water four or five hours in the forenoon, and three hours in the afternoon. Of course this kind of treatment would not suit English or Americans, but the place is well worth seeing. There are also single baths, but patients passing through so tedious a course of treatment would find it rather unpleasant to remain alone in a bathing-tub, for six or eight hours every day for several weeks. The time for bathing is from 5 to 10 a.m. and 3 to 5 p.m.

Visitors to Bad Leuk have the opportunity of making very interesting excursions to the neighbouring mountains and glaciers. I especially recommend a trip to the *Gemmi Pass* (2800 feet), where a grand view can be had of the various mountain ranges.

Hotels: Hôtel des Alpes, Bellevue, Hôtel de France, Union.

Physicians: Drs. Bonvin, Brunner, Grillet, Mengis.

Access: From London, Paris, Hamburg, or Bremen,

to Basle and Thun by railway, thence on the *Thunersee* by steamboat to Spiez, thence by carriage or diligence to Kandersteg, and thence on horseback to Leuk (bath) ; or from Paris, *viâ* Genève and Martigny to the railway station Louèche (Leuk) in the Rhone valley, thence by carriage to Bad Leuk.

PART III.

CHEMICAL COMPOSITION AND THERAPEUTICAL APPLICATION OF THE MINERAL WATERS.

GENERAL REMARKS.

EVERY patient visiting a watering place has a natural desire to know how the mineral waters operate on the system, and what are their active principles and curative effects. To satisfy this desire, I will endeavour to explain, in as popular a language as possible, the chemical composition and classification and the physiological and therapeutical action of those mineral springs which have been enumerated and described in the second part of this treatise, keeping aloof from all purely medical discussions, which instead of enlightening would only embarrass the mind of the reader. As aforesaid, this little book is written for the public, and not for members of the profession. For this very reason the comparative tables of the mineral springs, which will be found at the end of the book, will not contain *all* the mineral ingredients, but only the most important ones, the knowledge of which

CLASSIFICATION OF THE MINERAL WATERS. 175

will enable the reader to form an opinion of his own on the physiological and therapeutical action of the waters.

The following classification, based on the chemical composition of the springs, has been adopted by the best authors on balneology:—

I.—ALKALINE WATERS
1. Simple alkaline waters: Salzbrunn, Giesshübel, Neuenahr.
2. Alkaline muriated waters: Gleichenberg, *Ems*.
3. Alkaline saline waters (Glauber-salt-water): *Karlsbad, Marienbad, Franzensbad*, Elster, Bertrich, Rohitsch, *Tarasp*.

II.—SALINE WATERS
Baden-Baden, Cannstadt, *Homburg, Kissingen*, Nauheim, Pyrmont, Soden, *Wiesbaden, Kreuznach*, Münster am Stein, Hall, Reichenhall, Kreuth, Ischl, Aussee, Rehme-Oeynhausen.

III.—SULPHUR WATERS
Neundorf, Eilsen, Meinberg, Weilbach, Alveneu, Le Prese, *Aachen* (Aix-la-Chapelle), Burtscheid, Landeck, Baden (near Vienna) Baden (Switzerland).

IV.—IRON WATERS
Bocklet, Brückenau, Cudowa, *Elster, Franzensbad*, Homburg, *St. Moritz, Pyrmont*, Driburg, Reinerz, *Schwabach*.

V.—EARTHY WATERS
Lippspringe, Inselbad, *Wildungen*, Leuk, Bormio.

VI.—INDIFFERENT THERMAL WATERS
Schlangenbad, Warmbrunn, Wildbad, *Teplitz*, Johannisbad, *Gastein*, Tobelbad, Neuhaus, Tüffer, Römerbad, *Ragatz-Pfäffers*, Villach.

CHAPTER I.

ALKALINE WATERS.

Salzbrunn — Giesshübel — Neuenahr — Gleichenberg — Ems — Karlsbad — Marienbad — Franzensbad — Elster — Bertrich — Rohitsch — Tarasp.

POTASH and soda are alkalies. *Simple alkaline waters* contain soda in the shape of carbonate of soda, and a considerable quantity of carbonic acid. When either common salt or Glaubersalt is also present in a sufficient quantity to produce a therapeutical effect, the waters are called *alkaline muriated* or *alkaline saline* (Glaubersalt) waters.

Alkaline waters are colourless, perfectly clear, some tasteless, some with a salty taste, according to the quantity of salt they contain. Those rich in carbonic acid have a pleasant, prickling taste.

The most important constituents of the *simple alkaline waters* are carbonic acid and carbonate of soda. When drinking these waters, we usually notice an immense quantity of small bubbles; this is the *carbonic acid gas*, so well known to the reader as the principal ingredient of the common soda water. This gas acts as a stimulant on the stomach, and, if a moderate quantity be absorbed, also on the nervous system, producing lightness of the head and acceleration of the pulse and respiration. This latter effect is increased by a high temperature of the water. If too large a quantity of the gas is present in the water, part of it is soon eliminated by eructation. Waters with a small amount of carbonic acid are better borne by the stomach than those charged with a large quantity. To make the latter more digestible, patients shake it, or let the glass stand a short while in the open air, whereby the quantity of the gas soon diminishes. The presence of this gas, which increases the action of the stomach, renders all mineral waters more digestible.

Soda is present in the blood in the form of carbonate of soda or chloride of sodium (common salt), and its presence in the blood is of the greatest importance, as it keeps the albumen and fibrine of the blood in a state of solution, thereby promoting the assimilation. But the continued use of soda has a lowering influence on the system. Small doses of soda have a beneficial effect on the digestion. The prolonged use of large doses disturbs the appetite and impairs the nutrition. The excessive acidity of the stomach is neutralized by the carbonate of soda. This fact being generally known, many persons are in the habit of taking a small quantity of soda after dinner. Soda also increases the secretion of the urine.

The most striking effect of the alkalies is seen in catarrhal affections of the throat, bronchial tubes, stomach, &c. They promote the excretion of the mucous, and diminish its quantity. Experience has proved them, especially those which contain a considerable amount of chloride of sodium, highly beneficial in bronchial catarrhs; and their efficacy is materially increased by the high temperature, which aids the expectoration. Some of the alkaline waters are naturally warm, as for instance those of Ems, Karlsbad, &c.; others are heated artificially, if so ordered by the physician, or are mixed with warm milk or whey. Catarrh of the bladder is also benefited by the use of water containing carbonate of soda.

If the mucous membrane of the stomach is affected, carbonate of soda acts beneficially by removing the mucous and the gases, and by neutralizing the acidity of the stomach. There is hardly any disease in which more benefit is derived from the use of the alkaline waters than in chronic catarrh of the stomach and dyspepsia, the latter being in fact only a symptom of the former. Increased acidity, flatulency, copious secretion of mucous, and nausea, often combined with vomiting, are the principal symptoms. The digestion and assimilation being impaired, patients become lean and feeble. In all such cases alkaline waters, with the aid of a well-regulated diet, are the surest remedies to remove these symptoms. Of course no cure is possible without a rigid dietetic regimen, which, in each individual case, must be regulated according to the constitution of the patient and the prevailing symptoms.

Ulcerations of the stomach are also successfully treated by alkaline waters; but a careful supervision of the dietetic regimen is in such cases almost of greater importance than the use of medicine or mineral water.

In catarrh of the gall ducts, of which the principal symptom is jaundice, the alkaline waters, and especially the alkaline saline waters, are the proper remedies.

It has often been contended that alkaline waters increase the secretion of the bile; and there is some truth in that assertion, in so far as the large quantity of the water which is consumed by the patients increases the flow of the bile; the alkalies by themselves, especially the carbonate of soda, do not promote the secretion. According to Braun's theory, the Glaubersalt waters produce an irritation of the mucous membrane of the intestinal canal, and by reflex action, a stimulation of the liver, whereby the secretion of the bile is increased. At all events the fact cannot be denied, that a large number of patients who suffer from attacks of that fearful disease, gallstone colic, are greatly relieved, and often permanently cured, by the use of the alkaline, and especially of the Glaubersalt springs.

These waters are also very useful in cases of enlargement of the liver and obesity.

Scrofulous swellings of the lymphatic glands and thickening of joints improve by the use of alkaline waters, which greatly promote the absorption of all kinds of exudations.

Alkaline waters are the principal remedies for the cure of gravel. They prevent the formation of new calculous concretions in the kidneys and the bladder; however, those already in existence are not dissolved, as many believe, but are freely eliminated by the copious draughts of mineral water. Alkaline waters, especially when containing Glaubersalt, are very useful in gout.

In diabetes the alkaline waters, aided by a careful dietetic regimen, are the only remedy. I have seen a very large number of diabetic patients successfully treated by the Karlsbad waters; and, if the disease is not too far advanced, and consumption has not set in, the chances of recovery are favourable in the majority of cases. As the Karlsbad waters are almost a specific remedy for diabetes, this subject shall be fully discussed at the proper place.

A few words may be added, in regard to the action of *the Glaubersalt* (sulphate of soda), the most important constituent of the alkaline saline waters. It is present in the blood in a very small quantity, and has no specific physiological effect on the system. Small doses of Glaubersalt do not impair the digestion, but rather improve it; larger doses continued for some time impede the digestion, and produce dyspepsia, and catarrh of the intestinal canal; on the stomach and the bowels they act as a strong stimulant, increasing the peristaltic action, and causing copious watery purging.

Glaubersalt occurs in the alkaline waters in a comparatively small quantity, and combined with soda, common salt (chloride of sodium), and carbonic acid. This composition is a very good one, as the chloride of sodium and the carbonic acid stimulate the function of the stomach, and prevent the stronger Glaubersalt from acting injuriously on that organ. Glaubersalt waters have a mild, purgative action, without impairing the digestion; they promote the peristaltic action of the stomach, and enable it to eliminate its sour and fermenting contents ; moderate doses can be taken for a long time, without lowering the system.

Large doses, however, which cause irritation of the bowels and frequent copious ejections, act injuriously on the digestion and nutrition. It is generally known that moderate quantities of this salt, taken for some time, have a tendency to effect the absorption of the superfluous fat and reduce the weight, without any detrimental effect on the general health of the patient. Patients lay too great a stress upon the purgative action of the Glaubersalt waters, which, of course, is more or less powerful according to the quantity of water which they drink ; they generally labour under the erroneous impression that the curative effect can only be accomplished by large doses, which produce frequent, and even excessive evacuations.

Corpulent persons who wish to lose several pounds of their superfluous fat will find a sure relief at the alkaline-saline springs, provided they have sufficient energy to renounce the luxury of an opulent table, and to subject themselves to a rigid anti-fat regimen. Karlsbad, Marienbad, and Tarasp are the favourite spas of such patients. These powerful waters are also preferable to the other alkaline waters in cases of liver complaints, jaundice, hæmorrhoids, gall-stones, diabetes, gout, gravel, and chronic catarrh of the stomach ; they promote the circulation in the abdominal organs, regulate the peristaltic motion of the bowels, and by their purgative action relieve congestions of the internal organs. More shall be said of these matters when the therapeutical application of the various alkaline springs comes into consideration.

1. SIMPLE ALKALINE WATERS.

SALZBRUNN has two springs used for drinking, the *Oberbrunnen* and *Mühlbrunnen*, both cold (46°), which for nearly three centuries have enjoyed a great reputation as very efficacious in cases of consumption, bronchial catarrh, and catarrh of the bladder. On account of the high elevation, the place is more suitable for consumptive patients than its old rival Ems, whose warm climate and warm springs are too exciting for a large number of that class of patients.

GIESSHÜBEL : the principal source is the *Ottoquelle*, which, besides alkalies, contains carbonate of iron and a considerable quantity of carbonic acid. It is useful in catarrhs of the bronchial tubes and the bladder; as a refreshing drink it is in great demand at all the Bohemian spas.

NEUENAHR has four springs, all warm, like those of Ems, though not so rich in carbonate of soda. Temperature of the water 104° It is highly recommended in cases of chronic diarrhœa, bronchial catarrh, and diabetes.

2. ALKALINE MURIATED WATERS.

EMS, the oldest and most famous of the alkaline muriated waters, has six springs which are used for drinking: the far-famed *Kränchen* (96°), the *Kiesselbrunnen* (114°), *Augustaquelle* (103°), *Fürstenquelle* (96°), *Victoriaquelle* (82°), and *Kaiserbrunnen* (84°).

The great and well-deserved reputation of these waters depends on their chemical ingredients (soda, common salt, and carbonic acid), their temperature, and the mild climate of the spa; they are recommended—

(*a*) In catarrhal affections of the digestive, urinary, and especially respiratory organs, provided these organs be free from inflammation.

(*b*) In cases of vaginal catarrh and sterility. The *Bubenquelle* (96°), applied as an ascending douche, enjoys an immense reputation as a specific remedy for sterility, and is extensively patronized by ladies, and recommended by physicians, though this specific efficacy is doubted by gynecologists.

(*c*) The Emser waters promote the absorption of the exudations which often remain after pleuritic affections.

(*d*) In consumption these waters were, in former times, universally recommended by the members of the profession. Many experienced bath physicians now have a different opinion, and even forbid their employment in consumptive cases.

(*e*) Bronchial catarrhs usually derive great benefit at Ems; but if they are associated with hæmorrhage of the lungs, or with phthisis, these waters are considered injurious, such cases requiring a more tonic and invigorating air than is usually found at Ems.

Excellent whey of goat-milk, prepared by a Swiss, is very much used, generally mixed with the mineral water. There are also at this spa appliances for the inhalation of compressed air.

GLEICHENBERG has five cold springs (60°—64°)

which are far richer in carbonate of soda, chloride of sodium, and carbonic acid, than the waters of Ems. The *Constantin* and *Emmaquelle* are chiefly used for drinking, the *Roman-Karls* and *Werlequelle* for bathing. The *Johannisquelle*, which is two hours distant from the city, contains less soda and salt. The *Klausenquelle*, half an hour distant from the spa, is a strong chalybeate spring. The climate of Gleichenberg is far more suitable than that of Ems for patients whose respiratory organs are in a state of irritation. For this reason Gleichenberg is highly recommended for consumptive cases, and for all other affections which are treated at Ems.

3. ALKALINE SALINE (GLAUBERSALT) WATERS.

KARLSBAD has the only *warm* and *strong* alkaline waters of Europe; these are the most powerful of all the mineral springs on the continent, and deserve to be discussed more fully than the other waters. Their great therapeutical efficacy depends on the high temperature and chemical composition, combined with a suitable dietetic regimen. The high temperature facilitates the absorption of the waters, and alleviates the irritating action of the salt on the mucous membranes of the stomach and the intestinal canal; moreover, it increases the circulation of the blood, and the secretion of the skin and the mucous membranes.

The Karlsbad springs contain just enough sulphate of soda (Glaubersalt) to increase the peristaltic action of the bowels and cause evacuations without disturbing the digestion; if moderate quantities are taken,

ALKALINE WATERS.

which have only a mild purgative effect, the salts contained in these waters are absorbed, and operate on the system in the manner above explained, and this operation is soon noticed by the disappearance of the superfluous fat. Patients should therefore not urge their medical advisers to allow them to take large quantities of the water, or to give them purgative salts in addition to the water in order to increase its purgative action; because frequent and copious ejections are not desirable, as they would eliminate the greater portion of the salts, and thereby frustrate their absorption. One or two daily evacuations are sufficient for patients under treatment at Karlsbad. However, it is a general prejudice that a cure cannot be effected without much purging, and many patients feel unhappy, if they cannot daily register a considerable number of them.

Karlsbad has a large number of springs, which only vary in regard to temperature, their chemical composition being almost identical. The following are the most popular :—

        Sprudel 162°
        Neubrunnen 144°
        Felsenquelle 142°
        Schlossbrunnen 125°
        Mühlbrunnen 132°
        Marktbrunnen 124°
        Kaiserbrunnen 122°
        Kaiser Karlquelle 108°

The following table will show the quantity of some

of the ingredients and of the carbonic acid contained in sixteen ounces :—

	Sprudel. Grams.	Mühlbrunnen. Grams.
Sulphate of potass	1·430	1·450
Sulphate of soda	18·474	18·369
Chloride of sodium	8·002	7·901
Carbonate of soda	9·969	9·823
Carbonate of magnesia	1·279	1·239
Carbonate of iron	0·023	0·021
Carbonic acid	5·961	5·892

The water has scarcely any taste, some comparing it to a thin chicken broth; at all events, patients soon become used to it, and take it without any reluctance. The water of the Sprudel forms large incrustations; flowers and other substances, soaked for a time in the Sprudel water, are soon covered with a yellow or brown layer of stone, called *Sprudelstone*, which is a deposit from the water, and contains phosphate of lime, silicate of potass, and carbonate of iron. In the rear of the Sprudel colonnade, on such incrustations as protrude in the shallow bed of the river Tepel, visitors can observe a *green, sticky substance*, which is composed of confervæ and an immense number of microscopical animalcules. But the Sprudel water does not contain these animalcules.

The patient, after having taken two or three glasses of the water, notices a pleasant sensation of warmth through the whole body; afterwards, if some more cupfuls are drunk, a slight griping pain is often felt, and one or two evacuations are the palpable phenomena of the efficacy of the water. But this action does not always follow. At the beginning of the bath course constipation often annoys the patient, to his indescribable terror, for every one comes to Karlsbad impressed with the idea that the waters should operate at once, and produce an everlasting copious discharge of what he considers superfluous excremental matter. Such patients will undoubtedly be surprised to hear that invalids suffering from diarrhœa are cured by the use of the warm springs of Karlsbad. Generally during the whole course evacuations take place twice or three times in the forenoon. When the constipation continues, a small dose of Karlsbad salts will relieve the patient ; in such cases, it is often very advantageous to drink, before going to bed, one or two glasses of the water, which has previously been cooled. One of the most constant symptoms, is the increased secretion of urine, and the frequent desire to urinate. The perspiration is also somewhat increased, especially if the warmer springs are drunk. Eruptions on the surface of the skin, and increased secretion of mucous from the bronchial tubes, are also sometimes noticed.

The appetite is good, and often much increased ; a loss of appetite is sometimes felt after a prolonged treatment, but especially by patients who indulge in too large draughts of water.

The majority of those patients who adhere to a rigid diet grow thinner, while feeble persons who partake of a nourishing diet do not lose either flesh or strength. Diabetics who are ordered to eat much meat often gain flesh.

In consequence of the change of living and the scanty diet, patients often feel a little weak and languid a few days after beginning the treatment; but after a short time they recuperate, and feel lively and comfortable during the whole course. Some who are inclined to congestions of the brain, often feel a slight giddiness and dizziness of the head; but this disappears as soon as the quantity of the water which the patients drink is lessened, or if water of a lower temperature is taken. For a long time the prejudice has prevailed among laymen, especially in Germany, that a course of treatment by the Karlsbad waters, on account of their great efficacy, was a dangerous undertaking; and even nowadays quite a number of patients go there with a faint heart. *But there is not the slightest cause for such a fear, nor is there any danger whatever in the use of the Karlsbad springs, which I consider the most efficacious, the most beneficial, and entirely innocuous waters, if properly applied.* Of course patients often become worse during their stay at Karlsbad, but according to my own experience, based on several years' observation, mostly in consequence of their own carelessness in regard to diet, as a large number of visitors are too much inclined to disregard the simplest dietetic rules, and indulge in rather opulent or indigestible meals. This is the class of patients who loudly denounce these waters, as they are unwilling to confess their own folly. Furthermore, there are others who injudiciously take too large quantities of the waters, in order to enforce a rapid improvement; and others, again, who overtax their system by indiscreet active exercise. All these, and others who otherwise indulge in an improper way of living, cannot expect to experience a beneficial result from the use of the springs. I consider it my duty to urge this point, as patients who, by these and similar shortcomings, have left the spa without having been cured, are generally very apt to dissuade others from resorting to it, thus depriving them of the opportunity of recovering their health.

The monographists and encomiasts upon Karlsbad are in the habit of enumerating a large number of maladies which they claim as being benefited by the springs of that celebrated spa. I shall only specify those affections, which are generally acknowledged by competent authors as being cured or relieved there.

Karlsbad's waters are recommended—

(*a*) In *chronic catarrh* of the *stomach*, which the public generally calls *dyspepsia*. The predominant symptoms are:—Loss of appetite, pappy taste, coated tongue, bad odour from the mouth, acidity in the stomach, flatulency, eructation, nausea, and sometimes vomiting, whereby copious masses of sour, slimy substances are discharged. Patients also have a sensation of fulness and inflation in the epigastric region, often combined with pain and irregularity of the bowels; the nutrition is impaired, and there is a heavy feeling in the head and depression of mind. There exists hardly any other mineral water which has proved so efficacious and affords such a certain and often rapid improvement in these cases as the Karlsbad water.

(*b*) In *chronic ulcerations* of the *stomach*, where the Karlsbad waters are considered the sovereign remedy. The principal symptoms of this disease are the same as those of the former, combined with an intense pain in the stomach, vomiting after each meal, chronic constipation, and considerable emaciation.

(c) In *chronic constipation*, especially if caused by sedentary habits. The slow peristaltic action of the bowels, and the retarded circulation of the blood in the abdominal organs, are much improved by the use of the cooler springs of Karlsbad.

(d) In *enlargement of the liver*, especially if caused by an opulent table and want of active exercise. Patients of this kind will *positively* be cured at Karlsbad.

(e) In *jaundice*, which is caused by catarrh of the hepatic ducts. I have been informed by the oldest and most experienced practitioners of Karlsbad, that even the most pertinacious cases of jaundice are cured.

(f) In *gall-stone colic*. Very large quantities of gall-stones are often discharged without any pain by patients who drink the Karlsbad waters; and this is the first palpable effect of the treatment. But the principal object in view in the treatment of this disease is to prevent the formation of new stones, and this object is attained by an energetic use of the warmer springs, especially of the Sprudel. Patients who, by a first course at Karlsbad, find themselves relieved from the attacks of this exceedingly painful disease, should never neglect to return to a second course, in order to attain a complete cure, as the stones frequently re-form, and patients are only aware of their existence by the sudden appearance of a fresh attack.

(g) In *enlargement* of the *spleen*, which is easily cured, if caused by simple congestion and malaria.

(*h*) In *gravel*. Already in the beginning of the treatment numerous concretions often pass off freely and without pain. If the waters are taken long enough and in sufficient quantities, they prevent the re-formation of stones. The Sprudel is the most powerful and popular spring for cases of gravel.

(*i*) In cases of *gout*. This disease furnishes a very large quota of the visitors of Karlsbad, whose waters have a tendency to counteract the uric-acid diathesis, which is considered the cause of gout. There is no doubt, and the experience of many years has proved the fact, that the Karlsbad thermal springs are the principal remedies in the treatment of that disease. The best authors coincide in this respect.

(*k*) In *obesity*—excessive fatness, which is considerably and rapidly reduced at Karlsbad. Attentive visitors have ample opportunity of observing how much fat persons who attract attention by their immense corpulence are reduced, even within a short time after their arrival. Such patients lose twenty pounds, thirty pounds, and even more, within four or six weeks. But being accustomed to an opulent, rich diet, and unable to abstain from it after having finished their course, they soon regain their old weight. These are the patients whom we meet year after year at Karlsbad and the other alkaline saline springs—faithful and steady customers, anxiously longing every spring for the opening of the season.

(*l*) In *diabetes*. Four continental spas are recommended for the cure of diabetes: Karlsbad, Vichy, Neuenahr, and Tarasp, each of these having its special patrons and admirers among the members of the profession. The first-named seems to be the most favoured by the medical advisers of the diabetic patients, as the number of those who undergo a treatment at Karlsbad is very large, and increases from year to year. From all parts of the globe diabetics travel to that spa, confident of being cured by the far-famed thermal springs; and, indeed, this confidence is not misplaced, for the majority of patients find great relief. The symptoms of diabetes are generally known. An excessive thirst and hunger, very frequent discharges of enormous quantities of urine, loss of bodily strength, and great emaciation, are the first symptoms which attract the attention of the patient, and induce him to seek the advice of a physician. The examination of the urine demonstrates the presence of a more or less considerable quantity of sugar. The use of the Karlsbad waters, and a proper dietetic regimen soon effect a visible improvement; the excessive thirst and hunger diminish, the discharges of the urine become less frequent and less copious, the quantity of sugar decreases remarkably, and before the bath course is finished, the sugar often entirely disappears; bodily strength and hilarity of mind return, the bodily weight increases, and the progress of the disease is often arrested for years. Even in advanced stages of diabetes, an improvement is often attained, provided there be no complication with consumption or Bright's disease of the kidneys; cases of the latter kind are almost helpless, and no objects for treatment at any watering place.

In no other disease is the proper dietetic regimen

of such an utmost importance as in diabetes. Every violation of the dietetic rules, especially during the use of the mineral waters, is injurious. Having seen the most disastrous results caused thereby, I consider it necessary to designate the proper diet for diabetic patients, in order to enable them to select suitable food, as the bath physicians are often prevented, by the throng of visitors, from giving explicit instructions. The food should be prevailingly an animal one, and all substances containing sugar or flour must be rigidly avoided. Diabetics, who constantly feel hungry, should take frequent meals, and not eat too much at a time. For breakfast they are allowed to take coffee, without sugar or milk, a couple of eggs, a plate of soup, or a beefsteak. Milk should not be taken, as it contains sugar; cream is allowed. Bread is forbidden; but as most patients can scarcely do without it, they may eat one Vienna roll. *Kleberbrod*, bread prepared at Karlsbad for the special use of diabetics, is very useful, but patients soon become tired of it.

Dinner should consist of soup and meat—all kinds of meat being suitable—beefsteak, roast beef, veal, lamb, poultry, venison; the latter is very good for diabetics, and is always on the bill of fare at the better restaurants. Spinach is allowed, but no vegetables containing sugar or starch; as, potatoes, rice, turnips, asparagus, and fruit. Every kind of pie or pudding is strictly forbidden. Fish is a suitable food for diabetics; trout is the favourite fish at Karlsbad. Oysters, lobsters, crabs, are very good for diabetics; but not allowed during the time in which patients drink mineral waters. Eggs, in any shape whatever, are allowed ; salad, though a proper dish for diabetics, is not allowed so long as the mineral waters are taken.

For supper a plate of soup, meat, or a few eggs may be taken. One roll at every meal is all that is allowed by the bath doctors. To quench the thirst, patients can take a bottle of Giesshübel water, or a glass of red wine.

Diabetics being very liable to take cold, should always wear thick flannel underwear, and never take a walk without being provided with a shawl or an overcoat. Too much active exercise is to be avoided, as fatigue and exhaustion are injurious. To remain constantly in the open air when the weather is favourable, to stroll in the gardens or woods, is most beneficial to such patients.

Before closing the chapter on Karlsbad's springs, I should not forget to say a few words about the *Karlsbad salt*, which is extensively advertised and sold by the druggists of nearly every country of both hemispheres. It is a white salt, obtained by evaporation of the Sprudelwater ; 100 parts of it contains sulphate of soda 37·69, chloride of sodium 0·39, carbonate of soda 5·99, water 55·52. This salt has a well-deserved reputation, being very useful in cases of chronic catarrh and ulceration of the stomach, if taken in small doses; it is also applied in larger doses in all affections, where a mild purgative action is desirable. This salt operates quickly and without pain, and does not lose its efficacy like other purgative remedies, the doses of which must be increased from time to time in order to produce the desired effect. It has also another advantage above other purgatives, namely, while using it patients are not affected with subsequent constipation, which is usually the case after the application of other laxatives.

MARIENBAD has also powerful springs. The *Kreuz-* and *Ferdinands Brunnen* are strong Glaubersalt waters, and contain more Glaubersalt, chloride of sodium, and carbonic acid than the Karlsbad waters; their purgative action is also far more intense. The *Waldquelle* is a mild alkaline saline water; the *Ambrosius* and *Karolinenbrunnen* are alkaline chalybeate springs. All these waters are cold. The two first-named are applied in cases of habitual constipation, excessive fatness, enlargement of the liver, and congestions of the abdominal organs. They are eminently adapted for stout, full-blooded persons of sedentary habits, who, after having indulged in a luxurious, opulent living, are anxious to free themselves from their superfluous fat. For patients disposed to congestions of the brain, the Marienbad waters are better adapted than those of Karlsbad. The *Waldquelle* is recommended for chronic catarrh of the bronchial tubes; the *Ambrosius* and *Karolinenbrunnen* for anæmic affections.

Great importance is attributed to the peat baths, as has already been mentioned in the Second Part of this book.

TARASP.—Baun says, "The waters of Tarasp are in every respect a higher potency of Karlsbad and Marienbad." They contain the same amount of Glaubersalt, but three times as much carbonate of soda, chloride of sodium, and carbonic acid. Three springs—viz. the *Lucius*, *Emerita*, and *Ursus springs*—are strong alkaline saline waters; three others—viz. the *Bonifacius*, *Wy Quelle*, and the *Carola*—are alkaline chalybeate springs. All are cold springs. The purgative action is not too strong; but nervous excitement and sleeplessness are often noticed. Three to five glasses are the usual doses.

To stout persons, who have carried on an opulent, indolent life, the Tarasp waters will prove very useful. The magnificent mountain air, and the mild, equable climate, contribute a great deal to the success of the treatment, and give the place a great superiority over all other spas of the same class.

The waters of Tarasp are recommended for the same diseases as are those of Karlsbad, namely, for chronic catarrh of the stomach, fatty and enlarged liver, gall-stones, gravel, catarrh of the bladder, and diabetes. They are also highly praised for catarrh of the bronchial system, chronic inflammation of the uterus, and even for consumptive cases.

ELSTER and FRANZENSBAD have alkaline saline springs, called *Salzquellen*, which are similar to the Marienbad Kreuzbrunnen.

ROHITSCH.—The principal spring, called *Tempelbrunnen*, contains less Glaubersalt and chloride of sodium than the Karlsbad Sprudel, but more carbonate of lime and magnesia, and more carbonic acid. The water is cold, and is recommended for chronic catarrh of the stomach and of the intestinal canal, for chronic ulceration of the stomach, enlarged liver, gall-stones, gout, obesity, and especially for gravel and catarrh of the bladder.

BERTRICH has warm springs of 90°, which contain half as much Glaubersalt as those of Karlsbad. Its waters are very useful in cases of catarrh of the mucous membranes, gout, rheumatism, and nervous irritability.

CHAPTER II.

SALINE WATERS.

Baden-Baden — Homburg—Kissingen— Wiesbaden—Cannstadt—Nauheim—Pyrmont—Soden—Kreuznach—Münster am Stein—Hall—Reichenhall—Kreuth—Ischl—Aussee—Rehme-Oeynhausen.

THE principal mineral ingredient contained in the saline waters is the common table salt (chloride of sodium). These waters are clear and more or less salty, according to the amount of salt contained; if much carbonic acid is present, they have a pleasant, pungent taste. If the quantity of salt is small, say below two per cent, the waters are called *simple saline waters;* these are suitable for drinking and bathing. Some springs are cold, some hot. If the quantity of salt is considerable the waters are called *brines* (*Soolen*) and are only used for bathing.

There is a third group of saline waters, which contain iodide of soda or magnesia, or bromide of soda or magnesia; these are called iodo-bromate salt waters, and are used for drinking and bathing.

The saline springs are also classified, according to their temperature, into cold and thermal springs.

One of the most important constituents of these

waters is the carbonic acid gas, of which some of the saline waters contain a very considerable amount, which contributes largely to their efficacy.

Baths are given at all the saline baths, but while at some the drinking prevails, and only little importance is attributed to the bathing, the waters at others are so strong in salt, that bathing alone is practised. According to the prevalence of one or the other method, the saline waters are classified into *saline springs* and *saline baths*.

1. SALINE SPRINGS.

Small doses of saline water increase the appetite and improve the digestion, by stimulating the mucous membrane of the stomach and augmenting its secretion; the peristaltic action of the stomach is accelerated, and its contents are more rapidly removed. Small doses are absorbed, and improve the assimilation and nutrition. Larger doses produce watery alvine ejections, and, if continued too long, an irritation, and even inflammation, of the intestinal canal.

The active ingredient of these waters is the chloride of sodium, the *common salt*, which is the most important element in all organic substances. It is contained in large quantities in all tissues and liquids of the human system, and especially so in the blood, where its proportion is very large, compared to the other mineral constituents, as carbonate of soda, iron, &c. And it is to it that the saline waters largely owe their action. It acts differently upon the digestion from the carbonate of soda or Glaubersalt; for while these salts are *fat-destroyers*, and reduce the weight of the body, the use of the salt-springs does generally not affect the latter, nor remove a great deal of the superfluous fat.

As a constituent of all liquids of the system, the common salt is also present in the gastric juice, acting as a solvent on the contents of the stomach, especially on the albuminous and amylaceous substances, and thereby promoting the digestion and the absorption of the food.

Saline waters are therefore therapeutically applied when it is found necessary to increase the activity of the stomach and the intestines, to improve digestion and assimilation, and to promote absorption.

Carbonic acid is an essential element of all saline waters, the cold springs containing more of it than the warm ones. It is a valuable auxiliary to the chloride of sodium, as it operates not only locally as a stimulant to the secretion and peristaltic action of the stomach, but also, after absorption, as a general stimulant to the whole nervous system. This explains the pleasant, exhilarating effect of all beverages containing a large quantity of carbonic acid.

The *temperature* of the waters is also of great importance; cold waters are not so readily absorbed as warm ones; low temperature increases their stimulative action, while warm springs produce a sedative effect on the digestive organs.

The saline springs, especially the cold ones of Kissingen, Homburg, &c., have proved very beneficial in cases of *dyspepsia* and chronic catarrh of the stomach, when there is no complication with excessive acidity, in which case the alkaline muriated waters (Ems, Gleichenburg) are the proper remedies. Another frequent complication of gastric catarrh is obstinate *constipation ;* saline water could only benefit such cases if employed in large doses, which, however, would produce irritation of the stomach and of the alimentary canal. It is therefore advisable in such cases to resort to the alkaline saline waters of Karlsbad, Marienbad, &c., which are very efficacious in constipation. In chronic catarrh of the intestinal canal, the warm saline waters are very useful.

Patients of moderate strength, who are affected with hæmorrhoids, will do well to resort to a saline spring, while robust persons are more benefited by Karlsbad or Marienbad. *Congestions of the liver* and *fatty liver* are also objects of treatment by saline waters; but the Glaubersalt springs are far more powerful, and should always be preferred, if the disease is already in an advanced stage. In cases of *enlarged spleen*, produced by intermittent fever, the saline waters are employed with great success.

These waters have for many years enjoyed an immense reputation in cases of *scrofula*, and great results are undoubtedly obtained, especially by their external application in the shape of brine baths (*Soolbäder*). Swelling of the lymphatic glands, caries, rachitis (rickets), are successfully treated by the internal and external employment of the salt springs. Some of these which have a moist and mild climate, as for instance Soden, are highly recommended in cases of bronchial catarrh, and in the early stages of consumption.

The following are the principal saline springs :—

BADEN-BADEN : only one spring, called *Ursprung*, is used for drinking ; it contains thirty grains of common salt in one quart of water, very little carbonic acid, and has a temperature of 156°. Mixed with milk or goat-whey, it is recommended for bronchial catarrh. On the whole, there is not much stress laid upon the drinking, the spa owing its great popularity to its baths, its climate, and its magnificent situation and perfect arrangements.

CANNSTADT has four wells, which are used for drinking, and which furnish a mild, saline water, containing a moderate quantity of common salt and carbonic acid, and a small amount of Glaubersalt and iron ; temperature 60°—70°. In order to increase the purgative action of the water, sulphate of magnesia or soda is added ; whey is also mixed with the water. Three or four glasses of water, each containing about six ounces, are taken in the beginning, afterwards five or six. Chronic catarrh of the respiratory and digestive organs, and cutaneous diseases, are successfully treated.

HOMBURG has five cold saline springs, which are exclusively used for dinking ; these are, the *Elisabethbrunnen*, the principal source, which is richer than the Kissingen Rakoczy in chloride of sodium and carbonic acid, and a stronger purgative ; the *Ludwigsbrunnen*, *Kaiserbrunnen*, *Stahlbrunnen* and *Luisenbrunnen*, all of which contain carbonate of iron. The *Elisabethbrunnen* is the only water which produces copious evacuations and reduces the weight.

KISSINGEN has cold saline springs, which are rich

in carbonic acid and chloride of sodium, and contain a small amount of carbonate of iron. The two principal springs are the *Ragoczy* and *Pandur;* the third spring, the *Maxbrunnen*, is not so largely patronized. The two former have about the same chemical composition, while the *Maxbrunnen* contains only a small quantity of mineral ingredients, though it is rich in carbonic acid. The purgative effect of the Kissingen waters can only be attained by taking them in very large doses (a quart or more). They are employed in all diseases for which saline waters are indicated, and which have been enumerated above; they are especially recommended when the nutrition and assimilation are impaired, and the digestive organs relaxed, and not able to bear the stronger and more operative alkaline saline waters. In bronchial affections the *Maxbrunnen* is said to be very useful, taken either plain or mixed with wheys. The Kissingen *Bitterwasser* is used to relieve constipation.

NAUHEIM has two cold springs, which are used for drinking—the *Karlsbrunnen* and the *Kurbrunnen*, the latter being so rich in chloride of sodium that it must be diluted by some water in order to be fit for use; it is richer in salt than the *Ragoczy*, but poorer in carbonic acid. Half an hour distant from Nauheim is the *Schwalheim* spring, a mild saline water, very rich in carbonic acid, and chiefly used as a refreshing beverage.

PYRMONT, the celebrated iron spa, has also a saline spring, which is used for drinking, and contains about the same amount of chloride of sodium as the Kissingen Ragoczy, but less carbonic acid.

SODEN has an abundance of warm springs, all rich in carbonic acid and with a considerable quantity of chloride of sodium. The mild, sedative air of the place is exceedingly suitable for persons suffering from nervous irritability, bronchial catarrh, and tuberculous affections; patients, however, predisposed to congestions or affected with heart-disease should not go to Soden. The temperature of the twenty-four springs varies from 66°—156° F.; the springs are marked by the numbers I. to XXIV.; some contain chloride of sodium, others carbonate of soda and chloride of sodium; carbonate of iron is an ingredient of all.

The springs of Soden are especially recommended:

(*a*) For chronic catarrh of the pharynx, dyspepsia, catarrh of the stomach and the intestinal canal, chronic catarrh of the hepatic ducts.

(*b*) For chronic catarrh of the larynx and the bronchial tubes of delicate scrofulous persons, but not for those cases of catarrh which are associated with asthma of long duration, or with excessive discharge from the bronchial tubes.

(*c*) For those cases of phthisis where a temporary stay of the disease is noticed and the fever is subdued. Spring and fall are best suited for the treatment of such patients.

(*d*) For scrofulous and nervous women affected with chronic catarrh of the uterus.

(*e*) For nervous irritability, chronic rheumatism, convalescence after typhoid fever, scrofula, &c.

WIESBADEN.—Until the spring of 1879 only one spring, the *Kochbrunnen*, was used for drinking. A high temperature (156°), a moderate quantity of chloride of sodium, and nearly an entire absence of carbonic acid, are the characteristics of that spring. Its mild, sedative action on the intestinal canal, and the increased secretion of the skin and kidneys, are mainly due to its high temperature; moderate doses augment the peristaltic action of the bowels, and the secretion of all the mucous membranes; while large doses (a quart or more) effect copious alvine ejections, and diminish the secretion of the urine and skin. Such doses when continued for a longer time produce irritation of the stomach and the intestines, and congestions of the internal organs.

Catarrhs of the respiratory and digestive organs, especially when the mucous membranes are very irritable, are also benefited by the internal use of the Kochbrunnen. A new spring for drinking, the *Schützenhofquelle*, has recently been added. On the whole, bathing is by far the most important part of the treatment at Wiesbaden.

2. Saline Baths.

Salt baths have been used at all times; the Romans patronized them to a large extent, and wherever their legions were stationed, they searched for mineral springs and erected baths. They were acquainted with the saline baths at Wiesbaden and Baden-Baden, and used them extensively. Since the beginning of the present century a large number of saline baths have been erected at places where salt-mines were discovered and worked.

Saline baths are more numerous and more patronized than any other kind of mineral water baths. Besides the common salt, which is the principal mineral constituent, they contain chloride of calcium and magnesium, bromine and iodine, though these substances, on account of their small quantity, contribute but slightly to their efficacy. There is, however, another ingredient, which is considered a very important remedial agent in the external application of the saline springs, namely, the carbonic acid, with which some of them are highly charged.

The once general belief that chloride of sodium is absorbed by the skin, has made the salt baths so very popular, and even nowadays this opinion prevails among laymen. *But no salt is absorbed by the skin.* Nevertheless the common salt, aided by the high temperature, is the curative principle of these baths; and the experience of many years has demonstrated the fact, that saline baths are powerful remedies in various complaints. The salt acts as a stimulant on the cutaneous nerves; to this local irritation of the skin, by which the change of tissue is promoted and the circulation improved, the saline baths largely owe their beneficial action. If strong salt baths are continued for some time, the irritation of the skin becomes more intense, and often causes cutaneous eruptions. This irritation depends not only on the amount of salt present in the water, but even far more on the susceptibility of the skin; for there are patients endowed with such a sensitive skin, that even the mildest saline baths produce considerable irritation.

As above remarked, the efficacy of some of these

baths depends a great deal upon the presence of the carbonic acid. A patient immersed for the first time into water highly charged with this gas, is greatly surprised to find himself covered with an immense number of minute gas bubbles, which are spread over the whole skin, and look like innumerable little pearls —a very interesting sight. These bubbles are the carbonic acid gas; as soon as wiped off by the patient, they rapidly accumulate again on the surface of the skin. After awhile a pleasant pricking or burning sensation is felt, and a greater afflux of blood to the capillary vessels takes place, manifested by redness of the skin. Such a bath produces a feeling of warmth through the whole system. This sensation is due to the carbonic acid, which stimulates the cutaneous nerves, and through them the whole nervous system. To this action is no doubt due the great success of the thermal saline baths of Nauheim Rehme, &c.

The saline baths are classified into cold and warm (thermal) saline baths; those containing iodine and bromine constitute a third class.

The stronger saline baths are called *brine baths* (*Soolbäder*); a brine bath must contain at least two or three per cent. of salt. Saline baths which contain less salt are made brine baths by the addition of the necessary quantity of *Mutterlauge*, while baths which are too rich in salt are diluted by water, in order to avoid too great an irritation of the skin. The following table, showing the quantity of salt in the various waters, will be instructive to the reader :—

	Salt in 1000 parts.	Solids in 1000 parts.	Per cent.
Aussee	244·5	272·7	27·2
Ischl	255·26	271·6	27·2
Reichenhall	224·36	233·0	23·3
Pyrmont	32·00	40·4	4·0
Rehme	30·35	38·4	3·8
Nauheim	21·82	26·35	2·6
Kreuznach	14·15	17·6	1·8
Kissingen	10·55	14·2	1·4

Mutterlauge (mother lye) is a thick, brown liquid, the residue of saline water from which the greater part of the salt has been eliminated by crystallization. Dissolved in water, it is extensively used as a family medicine by the Germans, for the preparation of baths for scrofulous children. It still contains common salt as the principal ingredient, chloride of lime and magnesia, iodine, bromine, and sulphate of calcium. The quantity of salt in the Mutterlauge of—

Kreuznach, is 3·4 in 1000 parts.
Nauheim, is 9·3 ,, ,, ,,
Kissingen, is 56·0 ,, ,, ,,
Ischl, is 231·6 ,, ,, ,,

Saline baths augment the appetite, improve the digestion and assimilation, accelerate the circulation of the blood in the capillary vessels of the skin, increase the secretion of the sebaceous and sweat glands, and improve the nutrition of the whole body.

A most visible effect of the salt baths is the disappearance of scrofulous swellings. The success of the *external* treatment is much secured by the *internal* use of the saline waters, a method generally practised at the German spas. But however powerful be the action of these waters, we should bear in mind that the salubrious air of the spas, especially of those situated in mountainous regions, aids materially in procuring the beneficial results achieved by the *Soolbäder*.

There is also a great difference in the effect of the saline baths, according to the higher or lower temperature of the water, the cooler baths acting as tonics, the tepid ones as sedatives, while the hot ones are stimulating.

For therapeutic application the saline baths are recommended—

(1) In *rheumatic* affections and *gout*. The warm saline baths of 93°—95° have a beneficial effect similar to that of the indifferent thermal waters, which are usually applied in such cases; but the former being invigorating and strengthening, they are preferred in cases where patients are reduced in strength.

(2) For *atony* of the *skin*. Persons with a tender skin and apt to catch cold, are much benefited by cool saline baths.

(3) For *scrofula*. Saline baths, especially those containing iodine and bromine, are considered the real panacea for this malady. They improve the nutrition of the patients, and promote the absorption of scrofulous exudations.

(4) In *female complaints*. Chronic inflammation and hypertrophy of the uterus derive great benefit from the application of the saline waters.

The following are *mild saline baths*, containing one per cent. or less of salt.

BADEN-BADEN.—The temperature of the water varies from 112°—156°. The amount of salt contained in the springs being inconsiderable, it is the high temperature of the water that has made this spa so famous for hundreds of years. Pine-cone extract and Mutterlauge are used to increase the efficiency of the baths.

CANNSTADT.—The water has a temperature of 66°—70°, and a small amount of salt, but a considerable quantity of carbonic acid, part of which escapes when the water is heated for the baths; enough of it, however, remains to produce some stimulating effect. About 60,000 baths are given during the season. The climate is as mild and salubrious as that of Baden-Baden. Scrofulous and rheumatic affections, diseases of the skin and liver, are treated by these baths.

WIESBADEN.—The water contains only one-half of one per cent. of salt, and very little carbonic acid, but its virtue lies in its temperature, by which that great efficiency is attained which has established the immense reputation of this spa. The twenty-nine springs have a temperature of 142°—156°; but the water is mostly cooled to 93°, in order to make it fit for bathing purposes, and some quarts of *Mutterlauge* are added to increase its strength. Generally patients are advised to go to bed after the bath, in order to bring on profuse perspiration. Baths are given at the hotels, which is a great convenience for invalids, who are thereby enabled to bathe during the fall and winter without fear of exposure. Gout and rheumatism are the principal diseases treated at Wiesbaden, the mild climate being a great auxiliary in the cure of these affections. Persons slowly recovering from acute diseases likewise derive great benefit from the thermal baths of Wiesbaden, which are also very advantageous to delicate, scrofulous patients, who cannot endure a strong mountain air.

The following saline spas are *strong salt baths*, called *Soolbäder* (brine baths); some of them contain iodine and bromine, and a large amount of carbonic acid. At these places bathing largely predominates, though the drinking of the saline water is considered a valuable auxiliary, and much favoured at some, as at Kreuznach, Nauheim, &c.

.KREUZNACH, the most famous of the *Soolbäder*, owes its great reputation partly to the iodine and bromine contained in its saline water, which chemicals are popularly considered very efficacious for scrofulous swellings, and partly to the mild climate, the excellent arrangements, and the great perfection of the technical part of the treatment. The saline water is not strong, but by adding concentrated brine or *Mutterlauge* the required strength is readily attained. The internal use of the salt-water is highly praised by the Kreuznach physicians, and much practised, for the purpose of promoting the absorption of scrofulous swellings.

Kreuznach has four springs—the *Elisenquelle*, which is chiefly used for drinking; the *Oranienquelle*, the *Hauptbrunnen* of the *Theodorquelle*, and of the *Carlshalle;* the three latter being only employed for bathing. Patients, when entering on the bath course, take baths of fifteen minutes duration, but gradually the time of the bath is prolonged to forty-five minutes, or even to an hour. The temperature of the springs varies from 50°—86°, but for bathing purposes it is raised to 90° and 92°. The strength of the bath is gradually increased by adding *Mutterlauge*, of which even ten quarts are often mixed with the bath. Such strong baths, and the internal administration of the water, have a powerful effect on the absorption of scrofulous swellings; and the decided successes attained thereby maintain the high reputation of the place. Inhalations of the atomized salt-water are also administered.

All the different forms of scrofula are objects of treatment at Kreuznach, especially scrofulous affections of the glands of the neck and chest, and chronic eruptions on the skin. Scrofulous ulcerations of the bones, swellings of the knee-joint, inflammations of the eye and ear, resulting from scrofula, and rachitis, also derive the greatest benefit. Dr. Michels, of Kreuznach, especially praises the dissolvent power of the baths in cases of *tumors* of the uterus and ovaries.

MÜNSTER AM STEIN.—The principal spring of this spa, called *Hauptbrunnen*, has about the same chemical composition as the Kreuznach water, but a higher temperature (86°). The treatment is similar to that of Kreuznach. *Mutterlauge* and concentrated brine are added to the baths.

HALL, near Steyer (Austria), has five springs, containing iodide and bromide of magnesia; the principal spring, the *Thassiloquelle*, has a great reputation, and has been internally used since olden times as a remedy for struma. The *Mutterlauge* which is added to the baths, contains also iodide and bromide of magnesia; from six to twenty-five quarts are taken for a bath, mixed with the necessary quantity of mineral water.

REICHENHALL has a strong brine of twenty-three per cent. of salt, which must be diluted, in order to be fit for bathing purposes. The spa has nineteen wells, of which the *Edelquelle* is richest in salt. The temperature of the bath is 91°—95°. Patients affected with chronic catarrh of the bronchial tubes flock to Reichenhall, and are much benefited by the various remedies applied there, in the shape of inhalations of atomized salt water, compressed air, wheys, mountain bitters, &c., the fresh, pure mountain air being undoubtedly more efficient than most of these remedies. The brine of the *Edelquelle* is used for drinking, one tablespoonful being dissolved in a glass of water, but I do not think that much benefit is derived therefrom.

KREUTH.—The *Mutterlauge* used for the baths at Kreuth is carried there from Rosenheim, eighteen quarts being used for a bath. There is also a sulphur spring of 52°, called *Zum heiligen Kreuz* (to the holy cross), which is very much patronized by patients suffering from abdominal affections. Braun speaks very highly of this spa, and calls it one of the most wholesome watering places for irritable, scrofulous, and even consumptive persons, on account of the excellent mountain air and the good arrangements.

ISCHL has a strong brine of twenty-four to twenty-seven per cent. of salt. The bath is usually prepared with 100 gallons of mineral water, containing thirty-two to thirty-four pounds of salt, but it is often still stronger. A decoction of pine needles and some quarts of *Mutterlauge* are often added. Mud and vapour baths are also applied, and inhalations of atomized salt water administered. The mild climate is very suitable to persons suffering from bronchial affections or nervous irritability.

AUSSEE.—One hundred parts of the brine of this place contain eighty-three parts of salt. There are eighteen pounds of salt in a bath of about two hundred gallons of water, the brine is also used for drinking, though of course considerably diluted. Arrangements are also made for the inhalation of atomized salt water, pine needle baths, whey cure, &c.

KISSINGEN has two springs, which are exclusively employed for bathing, the *Soolsprudel* and *Schönbornsprudel*; they have a low temperature of 64° and 68°, and only one and a half per cent. of salt, and a great part of their efficacy is due to the large amount of carbonic acid. The *Mutterlauge*, of which from two to fifteen quarts are added to a bath, is rich in chloride of sodium. For the purpose of bathing, the temperature of the water is raised to 92°. Salt baths, of a lower temperature, but of short duration, are also applied by order of the bath physicians. The ascending douche, called *Welle*, and the horizontal douche, called *Strahl*, are very popular, the former one especially for uterine affections. Inhalations of atomized salt water, carbonic acid baths, peat and vapour baths are also accessories of this celebrated spa.

PYRMONT has a brine which contains three per cent. of salt, and a moderate quantity of bromide of soda and magnesia. Formerly the great reputation of this spa was based upon its efficacious iron waters, but for a number of years the salt baths have become largely patronized, and very beneficial results are obtained. The iron and salt waters are taken alternately or combined, as the case requires, and the existence of these two powerful remedial agents in one place is a great advantage.

REHME-OEYNHAUSEN has *thermal saline* water (brine) of 89°, which contains three per cent. of salt, and a large quantity of *carbonic acid*. Patients taking such baths should lie quietly, in order to allow the gas bubbles to accumulate on the skin, and produce the stimulating effect on the peripheric nerves. After the bath, moderate active exercise is recommended. Plain saline water baths (containing no carbonic acid) are also given in the *Soolbadehaus*. The *Sooldunstbad* (saline vapour bath) is a large domed inhalation-room where the saline water is atomized by falling down from a fountain of considerable height. The air of the room, which has a temperature of 87°, is very moist, and thoroughly saturated with minute particles of salt. It contains from two to four per cent. of carbonic acid. These inhalations are highly praised for chronic nasal, pharyngeal, and bronchial cattarhs.

Whey, the inevitable requisite of a continental spa, is also prepared at Rehme, and of course by a genuine Swiss.

The *thermal saline baths* (*Thermalsoolbäder*) are especially recommended—

(1) In *paralysis*. The splendid results obtained in

cases of paralysis have established the high reputation of the thermal saline baths. Bathing forms the principal portion of the treatment, the drinking being considered by competent authors as useless, and even injurious, as the exercise which is required in order to digest the water causes unnecessary fatigue to patients who need rest and recreation.

(2) In *spinal irritation* and *hysterics*. There is hardly any doubt that the thermal saline baths act beneficially, not only by the stimulating effect produced by the carbonic acid and the salt, but more so by the temperature, which is lower than that of other mineral baths, and therefore more invigorating.

(3) In cases of *protracted convalescence*, especially after typhoid, scarlet fever, &c.

(4) In *muscular rheumatism*.

(5) In *scrofula*. Rehme rivals with Kreuznach in the treatment of scrofulous diseases.

(6) In *atony of the skin*. The treatment consists in baths, whose temperature is gradually diminished. Great results are claimed at Rehme from this treatment.

NAUHEIM has three *thermal* saline springs (brines), which are used for bathing: the *Friedrich-Wilhelms Sprudel* (96°), *Grosse Sprudel* (89°), and *Kleine Sprudel;* the last one is at present used for carbonic acid baths. To increase the strength of the water, *Mutterlauge* is added.

These *thermal saline baths* (*Thermalsoolbäder*), which are very rich in carbonic acid, are applied for the same affections as those of Rehme. Professor Beneke, of Nauheim, praises their great efficacy in cases of articular rheumatism, especially when associated with heart disease, in scrofula, disorders of the uterus, and in eruptions of the skin, particularly eozema. Contrary to the opinion of other balneologists, Professor Beneke claims to have achieved splendid results from the treatment of skin diseases by mild saline baths, combined with the application of cold shower baths.

SODEN has also a *thermal* saline spring, with a considerable amount of carbonic acid, and a temperature of 86°. These baths act very beneficially on delicate scrofulous patients affected with bronchial catarrhs.

CHAPTER III.

SULPHUR WATERS.

Aachen (Aix-la-Chapelle)—*Neundorf—Eilsen—Meinberg—Weilbach—Alveneu—Le Prese—Burtscheid—Landeck—Baden* (near Vienna)—*Baden* (Switzerland).

THE peculiar odour emanating from sulphur waters has at all times attracted the attention of men, who being unable to explain the phenomenon, suspected something mysterious therein, and therefore attributed a singular power to these waters. Chemical analysis has demonstrated that the sulphurous odour is due to the presence of a gas called *sulphuretted hydrogen*, which emanates from almost all sulphur springs, though in greater quantity from the cold sulphur waters than from the thermal ones. This gas, though present only in a very small quantity, must be considered the principal effective constituent. Another gas, called nitrogen, and several mineral ingredients, as sulphate of lime and soda, chloride of sodium, and carbonate of soda, are also constituents of these waters. An organic substance, called baregine, is produced by decomposition of confervæ and algæ, which usually are present in sulphur waters. On the whole, they are nothing else but very weak solutions of those mineral constituents in water.

The most constant and most efficient constituent is the *sulphuretted hydrogen*. If carried into the blood through the lungs, or the skin, or the intestines, it soon permeates all tissues, but is soon again eliminated through the lungs and skin. This gas, when inhaled in a large quantity, is a strong poison; and even small quantities inhaled for a longer time produce a poisonous effect; when absorbed by the skin, it acts in the same manner. It destroys the muscular contractility; and muscular debility is a specific symptom of poisoning by sulphuretted hydrogen. When inhaled by the lungs, it proves sedative; the frequency of the pulse is diminished, and dizziness of the head, vertigo, and muscular debility are soon noticed.

Large doses of sulphur water produce analogous symptoms, the gas being absorbed by the capillary vessels of the stomach. It is also contended that this absorption produces turgescence of the skin, increased perspiration and secretion from the various mucous membranes and the kidneys. Sulphur-water baths retard the action of the heart and the respiration, and cause a feeling of comfort and ease. If the water is strongly impregnated with the gas, it acts as a stimulant on the skin, producing a pricking, burning sensation.

It appears from the experiments of competent scientists, that sulphur, carried into the system by the drinking of sulphur water, promotes the activity of the liver, increases the secretion of the bile, and accelerates the circulation in the large abdominal veins;

it therefore seems rational to resort to sulphur springs in affections of the liver, as for instance, enlargement and congestion, and in cases of retarded circulation of the abdominal vessels, which is considered the cause of hemorrhoids. Moreover, the liver being considered the principal receptacle of all metallic poisons, it is presumed that the sulphur by its specific action on that organ eliminates such poisons from the system. The efficacy of sulphur waters in cases of metallic poisoning seems to be generally conceded. Their operation on the skin is manifested by an increased turgescence and perspiration, and by a sedative effect on the cutaneous nerves; this action might perhaps account for the beneficial results obtained by sulphur waters in the treatment of rheumatism and several diseases of the skin. The secretions of the mucous membranes are also increased, and the tissues are relaxed; sulphur springs are therefore recommended as proper curative agents for chronic catarrhs of the respiratory organs.

Of the other mineral ingredients which materially contribute to the efficacy of these waters, the chloride of sodium is the most important. It is present in considerable amount in some of the sulphur waters, and is a valuable auxiliary, as it improves the digestion and assimilation. It is contended that those sulphur waters which contain this salt are the most digestible, and some authors attribute a large share of the success attained at the sulphur spas to the presence of that mineral.

The popular belief in *sulphur* and *sulphur waters* attributes the splendid results which undoubtedly are achieved at these spas, almost solely to the presence of that time-honoured mineral; but the quantity of sulphur in these springs being extremely small, balneologists express a less enthusiastic opinion of its therapeutic value. Braun, an authority in balneology, though not depreciating the efficacy of the sulphur springs, entirely denies their *specific* effects when *externally* applied, and compares their therapeutic action to that of the indifferent thermal waters.

The internal administration of the sulphur water is *en vogue* at almost all the sulphur spas; it is taken either pure, or mixed with milk, whey, or purgative salts. Patients commence by taking five or six ounces, gradually increasing the quantity to forty or fifty ounces; the cold sulphur water is often warmed, in order to render it more agreeable to the stomach.

The temperature of the baths varies between $92°$ and $96°$, a higher temperature ($105°$) being only applied at the celebrated Hungarian Herculesbad. The duration of a bath is from thirty minutes to one hour, and even three hours; one bath a day is the rule, but at some spas a bath is taken in the morning and another in the evening. Common baths for the simultaneous use of both sexes are still in operation at Baden (Austria), Landeck, &c. Ascending and descending douches are in general use, especially warm ones. The descending douches have a strong absorbing power, while the others, chiefly administered in the shape of uterine douches, are considered powerful stimulants. The vapour arising from the warm sulphur water is used for vapour baths, the temperature of which depends on that of the water; after the bath a sweat in blankets is usually taken. As these baths bring on a profuse perspiration, they are very valuable auxiliaries in the treatment of rheumatic and cutaneous affections.

Great stress is laid upon the inhalation of the sulphuretted hydrogen which rises from the surface of the sulphur water, and inhalation-rooms are established at most of the sulphur spas. The gas is inhaled either pure or mixed with other gases, viz. carbonic acid and nitrogen. These inhalations have proved efficacious in chronic catarrh of the throat and the bronchial tubes; but consumptive patients are advised to abstain from them, as hemorrhages of the lungs often ensue from their use. The inhalation of atomized sulphur water is also practised at many sulphur spas.

The most popular appliances at these places are the *sulphur mud baths*, which there are fully as much favoured as the peat baths are at other watering places. The mud is a deposit of the sulphur water, containing sulphur, sulphuretted hydrogen, and organic substances. Peat mixed with sulphur water, and impregnated with sulphuretted hydrogen, is also used. The temperature of a mud bath is about 100°, its duration from fifteen to sixty minutes. These baths are claimed to possess great curative power for stiffness and thickening of the joints caused by rheumatism, for paralysis, and especially for *sciatica*.

The sulphur springs are divided into cold and warm springs.

1. COLD SULPHUR WATERS.

NEUNDORF has three sulphur springs of 50°, containing a considerable amount of sulphuretted hydrogen, sulphate of lime (gypsum), and carbonate of lime; the water is applied in every shape—as bath, mud bath, gas bath, douche, and, mixed with saline water, as saline sulphur bath. The majority of invalids who visit the place are rheumatic and gouty patients; cutaneous diseases, syphilis, and mercurial affections, are also successfully treated.

EILSEN has ten sulphur springs, four of which are used. Temperature 53°. These are very strong sulphur waters, containing a considerable amount of sulphuretted hydrogen and sulphate of lime ; one of them, the *Georgenbrunnen*, is used for drinking, and then is generally mixed with milk. The mud baths, which enjoy a great reputation, contain much humic acid.

MEINBERG'S sulphur water has sulphate of lime and soda, and sulphuretted hydrogen, though less of the latter than that of Eilsen and Neundorf; the spa has also very efficacious sulphur mud. It possesses two springs, the *Alt-* and *Neu-brunnen*, which are very rich in carbonic acid ; the gas is used for inhalations and baths. Another spring, the *Schieder-* or *Salz-quelle*, containing a considerable amount of chloride of sodium and carbonic acid, is exclusively used for drinking.

The sulphur water, saline water, and carbonic acid are applied in divers combinations, and recommended for rheumatism, gout, scrofulosis, bronchial catarrh, and uterine affections.

WEILBACH'S sulphur water has carbonate of soda chloride of sodium, and a small amount of sulphuretted hydrogen. Temperature 56°. Owing to the presence of the alkalies the water is well digestible; it increases the appetite, and promotes the activity of the mucous membranes. It is highly recommended in cases of enlarged liver, hemorrhoids, and chronic catarrhs of the respiratory organs.

ALVENEU has a cold spring of 50°, which contains sulphate of lime, and a small amount of sulphuretted hydrogen, and is used for bathing and drinking. The high elevation of the spa, and the pure, bracing, mountain air, contribute greatly to the efficacy of the water, which is useful in cases of congestions of the abdominal organs, scrofulous affections, and bronchial catarrhs, &c.

LE PRESE has a sulphur spring of 46°, whose chemical composition and therapeutical application is analogous to that of Alveneu. The climate is mild, though the elevation is 3000 feet above the sea.

2. WARM SULPHUR WATERS.

AACHEN (Aix-la-Chapelle).—The thermal waters of Aachen contain only a moderate quantity of sulphuretted hydrogen, but a considerable amount of chloride of sodium, carbonate of soda, and sulphate of soda. This combination of salt is very important, as it renders the water very suitable for internal use. The high temperature of the springs and the most elaborate method of bathing are very important factors for the success of the treatment. The great reputation of Aachen as a sulphur spa is well deserved; thousands of invalids have been restored to health by the use of its springs; and notwithstanding the severe criticism of sceptical authors, the confidence of physicians and patients is unshaken, and the number of visitors steadily increasing.

The *Kaiserquelle* has a temperature of 132°, the other springs have 113°—120°. The considerable amount of chloride of sodium which is contained in the sulphur springs of Aachen, gives them a great advantage over other sulphur waters. The water is applied in every possible shape—as bath, douche, atomized water, &c. Vapour baths are also extensively used. The shampooing and kneading, which is an essential part of the treatment, is performed in a most thorough manner, and the douches are carefully and skilfully applied by the well-trained *doucheurs*.

The treatment of venereal diseases is a kind of speciality at Aachen, and great success is claimed by the bath physicians. But there are other diseases equally as much benefited, especially rheumatic and gouty affections, cutaneous diseases, paralysis, neuralgia, metallic poisoning, catarrhs of the throat, and bronchial affections.

BURTSCHEID'S waters are similar to those of Aachen.

The *Victoriaquelle*, which is used for drinking, does not contain so much sulphur as the Aachen springs, but the temperature is higher (142°). The same diseases are treated there as at Aachen.

LANDECK's springs contain a small quantity of sulphur and carbonate of soda. Two are used for drinking—the *Mariannenquelle* (71°) and *Wiesenquelle* (80°); three others forbathing. These waters are highly recommended for neuralgies (particularly of the face), and for uterine affections which are associated with congestions of the abdominal organs.

BADEN (near Vienna).—These springs contain a large amount of lime, and more sulphuretted hydrogen than those of Aachen. Their temperature varies from $79°$—$104°$. The *Römerquelle* (Roman well) is used for drinking, the other numerous wells for bathing. Scrofula, and catarrhs of the respiratory organs, are very much benefited; rheumatism, gout, cutaneous diseases, and mercurial affections, are also treated with great success.

BADEN (in Switzerland) has numerous springs, which contain only a small quantity of sulphuretted hydrogen, and of chloride of sodium and lime; but their temperature is high ($116°$). Twenty-one of them are used for bathing; the therapeutical application is analogous to that of the Aachen springs. Rheumatism, gout, metallic poisoning, neuralgies, and chronic catarrhs, are the principal objects of treatment.

The following table shows the amount of sulphur present in the above-mentioned waters:

Neundorf	0·0907.
Eilsen	0·0578.
Meinberg	0·0366.
Baden (Vienna)	0·0117.
Weilbach	0·0073.
Aachen	0·0056.
Baden (Swiss)	0·0025.
Landeck	0·0016.
Burtscheid	0·0007.

CHAPTER IV.

IRON WATERS.

Pyrmont—St. Moritz—Driburg—Elster—Franzensbad—Homburg—Bocklet—Brückenau—Cudowa—Reinerz—Langenschwalbach.

THE iron waters to a great extent shared the fate of the sulphur waters; once universally applied as a panacea for all sorts of incurable diseases, they gradually came into some disfavour with the members of the medical profession, especially with regard to their external application, though the belief of the large majority of patients in the magical power of iron was never much shaken. During the first quarter of the present century, the chalybeate springs were more patronized by physicians and the public than the other mineral waters; this was the period when bleeding was still very popular, and most extensively applied in every disease which was called by that ominous term *inflammation*. Bleeding was the first and indispensable remedy which had to be applied before all others; and every physician found guilty of neglecting the frequent use of that life-saving little instrument called the lancet, would have lost the confidence of his patients. Even nowadays bleeding is very popular in Italy, to the great detriment of the public; and it is positively asserted that the celebrated Cavour, the greatest statesman Italy ever had, perished in consequence of the frequent venesections, administered by his physicans.

By the liberal application of the lancet, patients who were fortunate enough to survive were so much debilitated, and so much impoverished in blood, the most essential element of the human body, that they repaired as speedily as possible to those springs which were considered infallible means of restoring *tuto, cito, et jucunde*, i. e. surely, quickly, and pleasantly, the quality and quantity of the blood.

Bleeding being almost entirely abandoned at the present time, the number of anæmic convalescents after inflammatory diseases has largely diminished, and consequently to a certain extent, the patronage of the iron spas. Nevertheless, there are always enough patients, especially of the fair sex, who are obliged to resort to them for the restoration of health.

There are some who doubt the efficacy of the iron waters on account of the very small quantity of iron contained therein. But experience has sufficiently proved their curative power; and though scepticism is the basis of all science and progress, we should not be too sceptical when practice demonstrates a fact which seemingly is not in accordance with theory. Small doses of iron *internally* administered, are able to produce a wholesome effect, and *iron baths*, though the non-absorption of the iron is generally conceded, *do act* highly beneficially; whether this benefit be obtained by the presence of the carbonic acid, or by the temperature of the water, patients do not inquire.

On the Internal Use of Iron Water.

Iron is an important constituent of the body, and of the nutriments which are consumed in order to maintain it. It is present in the blood, and its presence therein is of paramount necessity, the system being unable to properly perform its regular functions if the quantity of iron is much decreased. An adult has about nine pounds of blood, which contain from thirty to forty grains of iron. The muscles (popularly called " flesh) also contain iron, fifty pounds of muscle having about sixteen grains of iron. Our nutriments, especially meat, furnish the necessary quantity of iron we need for the support of our system. Animal diet, therefore, is very well suitable in cases where an increase of iron is aimed at, and a good beefsteak often operates far better than iron pills or mixtures. Suppuration, excessive secretions, especially diarrhœa, diminish the quantity of iron. The iron which the system receives by means of the food, goes to the blood, and is carried to the several organs; but a portion of it is eliminated by the secretions. The bile, for instance, which is richer in iron than the other secretions, leaves the body mixed with the passages, carrying off iron; urine also contains a small quantity of iron. If iron is administered medicinally, only a small portion is absorbed, while the larger part passes off as sulphate of iron, giving the fæces a black or greenish colour. The absorbed portion goes partly to the blood-corpuscles; partly to the several secretions. The system absorbs and assimilates only a certain quantity of iron, and cannot be forced to go beyond that—as many believe, who consume a large amount of iron in the shape of pills or mineral water; the superfluous iron is at all events eliminated, either by the intestinal canal or the other secretions. If the quantity of the red blood corpuscles is diminished, which occurs in anæmic persons, the internal use of small doses of iron augments their number. Iron waters contain only small quantities of iron, chiefly in the form of carbonate of iron; a patient in drinking thirty-five or forty ounces of the water in the morning, consumes only about half a grain of iron, which probably is absorbed; and during the usual course of four weeks he would consequently have assimilated about fourteen grains. Small as this quantity may seem, the case appears different when we take into consideration that the whole quantity of iron in the blood amounts only to thirty or forty grains, and that a loss of twelve grains suffices to produce a high degree of anæmia. It is therefore obvious that a gain of fourteen grains within twenty-eight days is sufficient to restore the blood to its normal state (Valentiner). This plain reasoning seems plausible, and probably explains the wonderful effects of the iron waters in cases of anæmia, which means *blood poor in iron*.

Iron waters improve the appetite, provided that the digestive organs are in proper condition; if the mucous membrane of the stomach or intestines is inflamed, iron water is not well tolerated. The latter acts as an astringent on the mucous membrane of the intestinal canal, and is often used with great advantage in chronic diarrhœa. It having been proved by recent experiments, that the internal use of iron increases the temperature of the body, it is evident that iron water should not be used in inflammatory or febrile cases; and the experience of bath physicians corroborates this fact.

Bicarbonate of iron being the principal chemical ingredient of the iron waters, its presence in a mineral water would make it a chalybeate spring, provided that the predominating effect of such a water be in reality that of the iron; for bicarbonate of iron is a constituent of a great many mineral waters, without however, having any visible effect, the other mineral ingredients being the real active factors.

Besides the iron, there is in most of these waters another, not less important and not less efficacious constituent, namely, the *carbonic acid*, which we have already mentioned in former chapters; iron waters are even richer in it than the saline waters. By its stimulating effect on the stomach this gas renders them more digestible; and by disguising the astringent and inky taste of the iron, it makes them more palatable. The stimulative action of the gas on the nervous system, undoubtedly increases the efficacy of these springs.

The temperature of the iron waters is generally low, ranging from 46°—64°, and must be raised for bathing. To avoid a great loss of carbonic acid, several appliances for the heating of the iron water are in operation, the best method being that of

Schwartz, according to which the water is heated by steam pipes running underneath the bathing tubs. For internal use the iron water is also often warmed, as many patients, especially young girls, do not well digest the cold springs.

The action of the iron waters is somewhat modified by the presence of several other mineral constituents, especially of carbonate of soda, chloride of sodium, and sulphate of soda. As the two first-named have a stimulating effect on the mucous membranes of the stomach and the bronchial tubes, the chalybeate waters which contain them will be successfully employed in chronic catarrhs of the respiratory and digestive organs; while those containing sulphate of soda are eminently adapted for anæmic patients, who suffer from constipation, or enlargement of the liver or spleen. Other iron waters, wherein lime is a prevailing ingredient, are beneficial in chronic diarrhœa.

Iron waters are almost exclusively recommended for that frequent malady of young girls, called *chlorosis*, in which the number of the blood-corpuscles is very much diminished. A pale face, bloodless appearance of the lips, general debility manifested at every active exercise, palpitation of the heart produced by the slightest bodily exertion, nervous irritability, and general relaxation, are the symptoms which alarm the relatives of the fair patient, and cause them to seek medical advice. Iron waters are the sovereign and never-failing remedy for this disease.

Anæmia is no disease in itself, but is a symptom accompanying various diseases, especially those connected with a great loss of humors, and signifies a deterioration of the blood, which is thinner, and poorer in red corpuscles. It is caused by hemorrhages, by prolonged suppuration of wounds, chronic diarrhœa, and similar discharges, which exert a debilitating influence upon the system. Such cases derive great advantage from the use of iron waters. Convalescents from typhoid and intermittent fevers, or inflammatory diseases, are also much benefited. These waters also render great service in cases of neuralgia, impotence, and enlargement of the spleen.

On the External Use of Iron Waters.

The time has passed when *iron baths* were considered the most effectual of all baths on account of the large quantity of iron supposed to be absorbed by the skin; nevertheless the majority of patients visiting iron spas adhere to that obsolete theory. It is always right to come out with the truth, even at the risk of producing an uneasy feeling; for unpleasant indeed it may be to many who strongly advocate the use of iron waters, to give up that long-cherished theory of the absorption of the iron by the skin. The harsh hand of science mercilessly destroys all prejudices and erroneous doctrines; and the absorption by the skin, be it of iron or other remedies, has for a long time been a favourite doctrine among physiologists, who could not otherwise explain the wholesome effect of a salt or iron bath. The most enthusiastic authors on iron waters do not at present believe in that dogma. Nevertheless, nobody would deny that these waters are strong remedies, and operate effectually on the system; but this action is solely obtained by means of the temperature and the *carbonic acid*. This powerful agent, whose action on the skin has been sufficiently explained in a preceding chapter (see Saline Baths), seems to be the most important and efficient element in the iron baths. The stimulating effect which it exerts upon the whole nervous system, cannot fail to enliven the whole process of nutrition and assimilation, and to promote the change of tissue. As plain water baths already have a similar beneficial effect on the system, this effect must necessarily be increased by the action of the carbonic acid; and competent authors have in fact demonstrated that chalybeate baths, rich in carbonic acid, far more improve the digestion and nutrition than common water baths. We are therefore entitled to define the external action of iron waters containing a sufficient quantity of carbonic acid, as one stimulating to the nervous system and aiding the change of tissue.

Patients when taking iron baths should keep quiet during the whole time they remain in the water; from time to time they may gently rub off the gas-bubbles which accumulate on the surface of the body; soon again innumerable bubbles will cover the skin, and a pleasant feeling of warmth spread over the whole system. To prevent the gas from escaping, the bathing tubs at some watering places are covered with blankets or wooden coverings. Half an hour's time is quite sufficient for a bath. Sometimes these baths cause head-ache, palpitations of the heart, disturbed sleep, &c.; if these symptoms of nervous excitement occur, the duration of the bath should be shortened to fifteen or twenty minutes, or the bath should be taken every other day, or diluted with common water.

The temperature of the iron bath need not be so high as that of the common warm bath, as the carbonic acid produces that feeling of warmth which otherwise is attained by higher degrees of heat. Therefore a temperature of 84°, which would be rather low for an invalid taking a plain water bath, is generally sufficient for a chalybeate bath. Such a bath has a tonic bracing effect, and patients feel quite comfortable while in it. For patients of great nervous irritability, or for those not possessing sufficient reacting power, the temperature may be raised to 88°.

We shall now proceed to enumerate the principal iron springs, the names of which are already familiar to those who have perused the second part of this book.

BOCKLET has one iron spring, very rich in carbonic acid and with an abundance of water. The bathing house has eighteen bathing-rooms, partly used for peat baths.

BRÜCKENAU has three springs, with a considerable quantity of carbonic acid and only a small amount of iron. Seven thousand baths are given during the season, one-third being peat baths.

CUDOWA has three chalybeate springs, the *Hauptquelle*, *Gasquelle*, and *Oberbrunnen*. Besides a considerable quantity of carbonic acid, they contain a fair amount of carbonate of soda and Glaubersalt, but not much iron. The spa has two bathing-houses with forty-eight bathing-rooms; gas, peat, and vapour baths are also applied.

DRIBURG has three iron springs, the *Hauptquelle*, *Wiesenquelle*, and *Kaiser-Wilhelmsquelle*, all containing a considerable amount of iron and carbonic acid.

ELSTER has six springs, which contain iron, Glaubersalt, soda, and carbonic acid. One of them, the *Salzquelle*, rather belongs to the alkaline-saline springs (where it has already been mentioned), the iron therein not being of much account, while the other five springs have a considerable quantity of iron, Glaubersalt, and carbonic acid. The *Moritzquelle* is the richest in iron, the *Albertsquelle* in soda, and Glaubersalt. Fifty thousand baths are given during the season, the fifth part of which are peat baths. Whey, that indispensable requisite of most of the Continental watering places, is also prepared.

FRANZENSBAD'S iron waters are similar to those of Elster—iron, carbonic acid, soda, and Glaubersalt being the principal chemical constituents. The quantity of iron is small compared to that of the salts, and hardly sufficient to effect a speedy cure in chloratic cases, but the large amount of carbonic acid gas renders the waters very efficient. Great attention is paid to the bathing, especially to peat baths.

The Franzensbad iron water is recommended for congestions of the abdominal organs, and especially for disorders of the uterine system when associated with an anæmic disposition. The *Eger Salzquelle* is an alkaline-saline water (already enumerated among these), and operates in the same manner as the similar springs of Marienbad. Of the other springs, which are chalybeate springs, the *Franzensquelle* is the most reputed; the *Wiesenquelle* is next in popularity, and the *Stahlquelle* has the largest quantity of iron.

HOMBURG has also a chalybeate spring, the *Stahlbrunnen*, which contains a large amounnt of iron and carbonic acid.

ST. MORITZ has two springs, the *Alte-* and *Neue-Quelle*. This spa has a predominant reputation as an iron spa, though its water contains only a moderate quantity of iron, and bears no comparison with the strong iron waters of Pyrmont or Schwalbach. But the presence of a considerable amount of carbonic acid, and the excellent pure fresh mountain air, will at all times insure for this place a prominent position among the chalybeate spas. In cases where the digestion and nutrition are much impaired, and in anæmic associated with great torpidity of the system, the water and climate of St. Moritz are of the greatest benefit.

PYRMONT, for centuries the most frequented and celebrated iron spa in Germany, has three iron springs (the salt spring has already been mentioned in Chapter II.). The water is one of the strongest iron waters on the Continent, and contains a very large amount of carbonic acid. Pyrmont has the advantage over other spas of possessing a first class iron and saline spring, alternately employed according to the requirements of the cases. The waters are eminently useful in anæmia, especially when associated with catarrhs of the digestive organs, in various nervous diseases—as St. Vitus's dance, nervous headache, hysterics, nervous debility, in disorders of the uterine system, in impotence produced by seminal loss, &c.

REINERZ has three iron springs, which are employed for drinking—the *Lauequelle*, *Ulrickenquelle* and *Kaltequelle*, the first being the richest in iron. There is a bathing house with sixty-three bathing-rooms, where 30,000 baths are given during the season; peat baths are also prepared. Diseases of the respiratory organs compose the majority of cases treated at Reinerz; but quite a number of patients affected with disorders of the digestive and uterine system also patronize the spa.

LANGENSCHWALBACH or SCHWALBACH has very efficacious iron springs, which are very rich in iron and carbonic acid, and contain a very small amount of magnesia and lime. There are seven springs, two of which, the *Stahlbrunnen* and *Weinbrunnen*, are used for drinking.

This spa is at present one of the most popular and most frequented iron spas on the continent.

CHAPTER V.

EARTHY WATERS.

Lippspringe — Inselbad — Wildungen — Leuk — Bormio.

MINERAL waters in which carbonate of lime (limestone), or sulphate of lime (gypsum), and magnesia are the predominant chemical ingredients, are called *earthy waters*, or *lime waters*. Lime is present in all tissues and organs of the human body; it is the essential constituent of the bones, in the form of phosphate of lime. We daily introduce a considerable quantity of lime into the body by means of our nutriments. All vegetable and animal food contains it; the meat we eat contains phosphate of lime in no insignificant proportion, and in all the water we drink lime is also present. Thus it is evident that lime is furnished by the food in sufficient quantity for the support of the body.

In mineral waters lime occurs as carbonate and sulphate of lime; the latter being indigestible, most of it passes off through the alimentary canal; a portion of the carbonate of lime is absorbed if the mineral water is taken on an empty stomach; the rest passes off with the alvine excretions. In what manner the carbonate of lime acts on the system, we cannot sufficiently explain. The carbonate of lime and magnesia, when taken in small doses, are well borne by the stomach; as they neutralize the acids of the gastric juice, they are often applied in irregularities of the digestion caused by excessive acidity. Lime retards the action of the bowels and checks diarrhœa; carbonate of magnesia acts as a mild aperient when taken in large doses.

There exists a disease of children, called *rachitis* (rickets), which is caused by a deficiency of lime in the bones, and for a long time the extensive internal application of lime water was considered an infallible remedy for it. But there is some error in this theory, as too large quantities of lime employed for the cure of rachitis are of no value at all; for the cause of the disease is not that too small a quantity of lime is *consumed* by the little patients, but that too small a quantity is *absorbed* and *assimilated*, the stomach of the patient not being in proper working order, and unable to absorb the necessary quantity. As long as this deficiency exists, it is evidently useless to overload the digestive apparatus with huge draughts of lime water, of which the greater portion would pass off without any benefit to the patient. In such cases small doses are profitable, in order to neutralize the acidity and augment the activity of the stomach.

Lime has an astringent and exsiccating effect on the mucous membranes; it is therefore not only used in profuse secretions of the alimentary canal (in diarrhœa), but also in excessive secretions of the bronchial tubes and catarrhs of the genito-urinary system.

In addition to lime and magnesia, the earthy waters contain a small quantity of common salt, and more or less iron and carbonic acid.

These waters are profitably employed as baths; but as neither lime nor magnesia is absorbed by the skin, it is presumed that their efficacy, when externally applied, rests with their temperature and the carbonic acid.

Earthy waters are recommended in cases of rachitis, anæmia, scrofula, gravel, catarrh of the bladder and the respiratory organs.

Of all the spas mentioned in our topographical review, only five belong to the class of the earthy waters, namely, Lippspringe, Inselbad, Wildungen, Leuk, Bormio.

LIPPSPRINGE.—Its principal spring, the *Arminius-quelle*, enjoys a very great reputation, and contains limestone, gypsum, and a small amount of iron; the gases emanating from the spring are composed of eighty-seven per cent. nitrogen and thirteen per cent. carbonic acid. Great stress is laid upon the inhalation of these gases, which are praised as very effectual in consumption, catarrh of the throat and bronchial tubes, and in asthma. The nitrogen is pretended to have a sedative effect, while the carbonic acid is exciting. It is asserted that consumptive patients while inhaling the gaseous moist air feel comfortable and relieved, that the respiration becomes freer and deeper, that the irritation of the mucous membrane, which causes the troublesome cough, is appeased, and the frequency of the pulse diminished; even neuralgic pains are soon relieved. There seems to be no doubt that the water of Lippspringe and the inhalation of the nitrogen are very wholesome for catarrhs of the larynx and the bronchial tubes; their efficacy in the early stages of consumption has been proved, according to the reports of experienced bath physicians, in a very large number of cases, and we cannot question the veracity of scientific men, who base their accounts upon the observations of many years.

INSELBAD has three springs—the *Ottilienquelle*, which is richer in nitrogen and chloride of sodium than the Arminiusquelle at Lippspringe, the *Badequelle*, of the same chemical composition as the former, and the *Marienquelle*, an iron water with a considerable amount of bicarbonate of iron (0·058). There are two inhalation-rooms, where the nitrogen emanating from the *Ottilienquelle* is inhaled by patients suffering from affections of the lungs. As this spring has less carbonic acid than the Arminiusquelle, it is less exciting, and acts more sedative. Several apparatuses for the inhalation of the *atomized* water are in the same rooms. Diseases of the larynx and the lungs are the specialties treated at this place. The large swimming bath and the use of the iron water are very suitable for convalescents and anæmic patients.

WILDUNGEN has numerous springs, of which only five are used, all very rich in carbonic acid. Besides lime and magnesia, they contain carbonate of iron. The *Helenenquelle*, *Königsquelle*, and *Georg Victorsquelle* are the most popular. Wildungen's waters have an immense reputation as a specific for catarrh of the bladder, swelling of the prostatic gland, and gravel; they are also useful in catarrh of the stomach and the intestines, anæmia, and general debility.

LEUK has twenty-two springs. The Lorenzquelle, which is used for drinking, contains limestone, gypsum, and a small amount of carbonic acid. Its action on the bowels is astringent and constipating. The rigid method of bathing, as applied at Leuk in the shape of immersions of several hours' duration, is undoubtedly very apt to produce favourable results in chronic diseases of the skin, especially eczema and psoriasis, and in cases of thickenings of the joints, which so often accompany rheumatic and gouty affections. For a long time protracted warm water baths have been employed with great success by Hebra, the greatest living authority in dermatology. It seems obvious that the similar method applied at the warm mineral springs of Leuk, aided by the fresh, bracing mountain air of 4400 feet elevation, should also prove highly advantageous. A skin thoroughly macerated by long-continued immersions must necessarily throw off the old, diseased layers, and form new ones, a process by which alone inveterate cases may be permanently cured. By the same method, old atomic ulcerations of the leg are successfully treated.

BORMIO possesses eight springs, which supply the old and new baths, and also furnish a muddy deposit, consisting of mineral ingredients and algae, used for mud baths. The water is poor in mineral ingredients, and poorer still in carbonic acid. But its high temperature ($102°$), the beautiful situation of the place, the fresh, invigorating mountain air, are certainly apt to prove beneficial in all such affections, which generally are successfully treated by warm mineral waters, as rheumatism, gout, neuralgia, paralysis caused by suppressed perspiration of the skin, and divers female disorders.

The application of mud baths materially aids the efficacy of the thermal waters.

CHAPTER VI.

INDIFFERENT THERMAL WATERS.

Schlangenbad—Wildbad—Gastein—Teplitz—Ragatz· Pfäffers—Johannisbad—Warmbrunn—Tobelbad —Neuhaus—Tüffer—Römerbad—Villach.

A LARGE number of thermal waters occur in every part of the globe. They are called *indifferent thermal waters*, on account of the insignificant quantity of mineral constituents which they contain; but the reader should not on that account infer that they are of little therapeutic value. By no means; for the high temperature of these springs, and the salubrious air, exert a very beneficial influence on many chronic diseases. For a long time these waters were much neglected by physicians, who judge the efficacy of a mineral water solely by its chemical composition; but they were restored to their proper rank among the mineral springs by experienced physicians, who, by careful and critical observation, proved their unquestionable curative effects, especially in many nervous affections. These effects are so striking, that the late Professor Romberg, of Berlin, one of the most celebrated neurologists, was wont to denominate these baths *nerve-baths*. In Germany they are often called *Wildbäder* (wild baths), as they are generally situated in wild, wooded, and hilly regions, some even on high Alpine heights. For two or three decades the indifferent thermal baths have become exceedingly popular, and the majority of them are crowded in the height of the season.

As the temperature seems to be the only curative agent of these waters, some practitioners believe that common water, raised to the required heat, would have the same curative effect as have the indifferent thermal springs. But those who are acquainted with the latter through personal experience have come to a quite different conclusion. An attentive bather, when immersing himself into a thermal bath, will notice a very pleasant sensation, quite different from the one experienced in an artificially heated bath. This is no imagination, for experience has proved the superiority of the thermal baths. By what agency this pleasant sensation is produced cannot be stated; nowadays we do not believe in that mysterious *Brunnengeist* (spirit of the well) of olden times, which was considered the invisible agent by which were accomplished those wonderful cures so often attained at these springs.

The thermal water is clear, transparent, and odourless; in a large basin with a white bottom it presents a greenish appearance. Immersed into this water the patient experiences a delightful feeling of repose and comfort, and a very agreeable sensation of smoothness upon passing the hand over the skin. The water is soft and mild on account of the absence of salt and carbonic acid; nitrogen and oxygen are present in considerable quantities.

At some of the indifferent spas, the practice of drinking the thermal water is indulged in, although probably without any other effect than that of large draughts of warm water, i. e. that of diluting the contents of the stomach and the intestines, and increasing the secretions of the skin and the kidneys. The peristaltic action of the bowels is also gently promoted.

But no importance is generally attached to the drinking, bathing being almost the only and all important business at the *Wilbäder*. The effects of the baths vary according to the lower or higher temperature of the water. Baths are taken either lukewarm or hot; the temperature of the former varies from 90°—94°, and has no influence on the natural warmth of the body, which remains the same, no matter how long the bath may last. The lukewarm thermal bath increases the activity of the skin, and acts as a sedative on the cutaneous nerves; the morbid irritability of the nerves decreases, and a feeling of quiet and comfort takes place. Such tepid thermal baths are therefore especially styled *nerve-baths*, and much patronized as such. Among them Schlangenbad takes the lead; Johannisbad, Tabelbad, and Villach, belong to the same class. The pleasant location of these baths in quiet and picturesque regions, surrounded by woods and mountains, cannot be too highly appreciated, as such environs act in a calming, quieting manner on the mind of the patients, and aid the sedative action of the thermal water. Bath life at these spas is also generally a quiet one, and therefore very well suited for nervous persons.

The hot baths at the indifferent springs have a temperature of 96°—106°. They increase the natural temperature of the body, accelerate the circulation of the blood, and produce a flow of the latter to the capillary vessels of the skin, causing thereon hyperæmia, redness, and increased perspiration. *Heat is motion*, according to the doctrines of natural philosophy; when the heat of the body is augmented, the smallest particles of the latter are set in a quicker motion. By this increased motion the adhesion of these minute molecules (atoms) is impaired, and the molecular attraction decreases. It is contended that such a process is produced by the hot thermal-baths, and the resolution and absorption of exudations is thereby perfected. This plausible theory is very well adapted to explain the splendid results achieved by the hot springs of Teplitz, Gastein, &c., in rheumatic exudations and similar affections. The effect of the hot bath is an exciting one, the irritability of the nervous system being increased. In consequence of the accelerated circulation of the blood and the greater fulness of the blood vessels, there is great danger of congestions of the internal organs, especially of the brain and heart. Persons predisposed to congestions, or affected with diseases of the heart, should therefore not take hot baths.

The best time for bathing is in the early morning, and with an empty stomach, provided the patient be not too much debilitated. After the bath, a short rest is advisable; rheumatic and gouty patients would do well to go to bed and take a good sweat in blankets. Those afflicted with neuralgia or paralysis, should avoid further perspiration after the bath; to keep cool and take a little walk, will suit them better.

It is the rule to take a bath every day, but weak persons should bathe only every other day.

Douches and shower baths are employed at most of the spas, and contribute a great deal to the success of the treatment. They are powerful remedies, if properly applied, and should not be trifled with, as their injudicious application often proves very injurious. Patients should follow the advice of bath physicians, and not allow the attendants to apply the douches *ad libitum*.

Long experience and careful observation have indicated the cases which are profitably treated at the thermal spas. Chronic rheumatism of the joints, as well as of the muscles, and gout, are the diseases which furnish the largest contingent to the army of patients who crowd these places every season, seeking and finding relief from their ailments. Gun-shot wounds, ulcers with unhealthy suppuration, stiffness of the joints after fractures or luxations, are also very much benefited.

Exudations which often remain after inflammatory diseases, are brought to absorption by the indifferent waters.

The diseases of the nervous system are also proper objects of treatment, but there is a great difference in the operation of the various springs. If great irritability of the nervous system is the cause of the disease, as is the case in hysterical affections, nervous headache, sleeplessness, spinal irritation, St. Vitus's dance, and in many forms of neuralgia, the cooler indifferent waters of Schlangenbad, Johannisbad, &c., should be resorted to; in all forms of paralysis, be they caused by affections of the brain or spine, the hotter springs of Teplitz, Gastein, &c., should be chosen. A large number of uterine affections are also treated with great success at some of these spas; Schlangenbad has a special reputation with regard to these irregularities.

Diseases of the skin, metallic poisoning, and general debility after acute diseases, are also cured by the indifferent waters.

The following are the most popular of the indifferent thermal springs.

SCHLANGENBAD is at present the best patronized of the cooler *Wildbäder*. Its waters have a temperature of 82°—92°, and are highly praised for their quieting and invigorating action on the nervous system. All kinds of nervous affections are treated, the spa being the greatest favourite with the ladies. The place has three bathing-houses with douches, &c. Fresh iron water is carried thither every day from Schwalbach and used by the patients; whey, milk, grape, and herb-cures are also very popular.

JOHANNISBAD has an abundance of water of 86°, belonging to the class of the cooler thermal spas; it much resembles Schlangenbad, and has a similar calming and invigorating effect; the pure, bracing forest and mountain air is a great advantage of the place.

TABELBAD has a water of 87°, the effect of which is similar to that of the above-named springs.

VILLACH has an abundance of clear thermal water of 84°, which supplies two large swimming baths, and quite a number of single baths and douches.

TEPLITZ, the foremost of the *Wildbäder*, has an abundance of water, the temperature of which ranges from 86°—118°. A short time ago, the inhabitants of this old, celebrated spa were terrified by the sudden disappearance of the principal well, caused by an accident which befell the mines of the neighbouring city of Dux. But happily their anxiety was soon relieved by prompt action of the authorities, and the salutary springs again flow as copiously as ever.

The waters of Teplitz take the lead among the hot thermal springs; they have an exciting, stimulating effect, and are employed with the greatest advantage in cases of rheumatism, gout, paralysis, &c.

On account of the great throng of visitors, patients are obliged to commence bathing very early in the morning, and those who neglect to engage a bathing-room at the proper time, will find it difficult to be accommodated in the height of the season. A new bathing-house for the use of peat baths has lately been erected.

GASTEIN resembles Teplitz in point of high temperature of the water, which varies from 96°—118°. Its springs are exceedingly beneficial for the same affections which are cured at Teplitz, but owing to the high elevation and the fresh, invigorating Alpine air of Gastein, weak and irritable patients can endure the high temperature of the water better than they would at Teplitz, which has a warmer climate. Less irritable and stronger patients may resort to the latter spa.

RAGATZ-PFÄFFERS has the advantage over Gastein of easy access by railway. The temperature of the water is 94°—99°. Gout, rheumatism, and paralysis are successfully treated. Whey and grape cures are also practised.

WILDBAD ranks next to Teplitz in regard to popularity and frequency. The water has a temperature of 93°—98°; two of the springs are used for drinking. The same diseases are treated there as at the other indifferent spas. The inevitable whey is also prepared and much patronized.

WARMBRUNN has four springs, with a temperature of 96°—108°. Gouty and rheumatic patients derive great benefit from the use of these waters.

NEUHAUS, TÜFFER and RÖMERBAD have waters a temperature of 95°—102°. These spas are visited by patients suffering from the same diseases as those who throng the other more celebrated *Wildbäder*. They are also very much recommended for hysterics and uterine complaints.

PART IV.

CLIMATOLOGICAL AND BALNEOLOGICAL NOTES.

CHAPTER I.

CLIMATIC HEALTH RESORTS, WITH SPECIAL REFERENCE TO PULMONARY CONSUMPTION.

CHANGE of air has at all times been considered one of the most important curative agents in chronic diseases. Patients suffering from rheumatic or nervous affections, from bronchial catarrhs, scrofula, and other ailments, have found, and will always find relief, or complete restoration to health, by changing the cold northern climate, which is so unfavourable for the cure of a great number of chronic affections, for the mild, warm air of southern regions. The observation made by experienced practitioners, that many chronic diseases take a more favourable course during the warm season, has always induced them to send patients for the fall and winter to a southern country, where they may enjoy, even during those seasons, the advantages of a warm, equable climate, and constant outdoor exercise.

Physicians have at last come to the conclusion, that fresh air alone is the real elixir of life for many complaints, especially pulmonary ones. The time has passed when practitioners believed in curing pulmonary consumption by large bottles of medicine, when the stomach of the unfortunate victim was made a depository for all kinds of drugs, or when desponding physicians, terrified by the first symptoms of that abominable evil which decimates the human race, left the patients to their mournful fate, considering them hopeless from the beginning. Medical science having demonstrated that incipient phthisis *can* be cured, it is the duty of a conscientious medical adviser to discover, by a scrupulous examination, the first symptoms of the disease, and to take proper steps in order to arrest its further progress.

Suspicion of pulmonary consumption should always be aroused when persons of consumptive parents, or those whose sanitary surroundings are bad, apply for medical advice.

Bad air is the principal factor in the generation of disease, and natural science has already almost established the hypothesis, that many diseases are produced by germs floating in the atmosphere. Upon this hypothesis the great English surgeon, Mr. Lister, has based his new method of antiseptic treatment of wounds, destroying, by means of carbolic acid, the germs in the immediate vicinity of wounds—a method by which thousands of lives have been saved after operation.

Some eminent scientists have expressed the opinion, that pulmonary consumption also generates by germs, and as city air is particularly contaminated by them, it is evident that a change of residence will prove highly beneficial to all those who live in large overcrowded cities. City air is poisoned by smoke, obnoxious gases, and especially by dust; the latter contains incalculable quantities of pernicious substances, particularly such as arise from the refuse of houses and factories. Tyndall has demonstrated that the atmospheric dust of our rooms is almost exclusively composed of organic substances. It is obvious that such a contaminated air is injurious to any patient, but particularly to a consumptive one, and that change of air should be the first condition when a treatment is commenced. However, the air should not only be free from impurities, but also of a temperature suitable to phthisical patients, who, in order to derive a real benefit from the change of residence, should be constantly in the open air. Experience has proved that persons who spend their time almost constantly outdoors and in a pure air, as for instance nomads, hunters, mountaineers, and others of similar habits, are rarely affected with consumption. It is reported that the Kirghises, who live a nomadic life on the Russian steppes, enjoy a perfect immunity from phthisis; it is also a fact that persons born and reared on elevated regions, and who while living in cities are attacked by pulmonary complaints, soon recover on returning to the mountains. Although the immunity from consumption claimed for Alpine regions is not so unquestionably proved as the enthusiastic friends of elevated regions contend, we must nevertheless acknowledge that phthisis does not so frequently occur in high elevations as in the plains; and that patients, if under proper treatment, greatly improve by a sojourn in mountain regions. This experience has led to the erection of sanitariums at elevated points.

The advantages of a stay on Alpine heights result from various circumstances, as, insulation, temperature, evaporation, freshness and purity of air, &c. The sunlight is more intense on high mountains, particularly in summer, and the atmosphere drier, than that of the lower plains. The temperature, on the contrary, decreases in proportion to the elevation, and the cool, fresh air is apparently the principal factor of the beneficial influence exerted by the Alpine climate on phthisical patients. Furthermore, by the change from the air of the plains to that of the mountains, the appetite increases, the nutrition and assimilation improve, and the fresh air, which is entirely free from the dust and emanations of the city, acts really regenerative upon the whole system. The scanty population of high regions is also a very favourable circumstance, for it cannot be denied that the crowding of a large number of human beings in a comparatively small, circumscribed place, is one of the principal causes in the production of disease, and thus our large cities are the breeding places of consumption and other allied maladies.

But patients should not believe that a residence at one of the health-stations, be it on Alpine heights or in more southern regions, is all that is necessary to perfect a cure; this alone is not sufficient. One of the first and indispensable requisites, wherever the patients sojourn, is a strict medical supervision, and next to that such complete arrangements of living as patients suffering from a severe disease require. The most salubrious climate, and the purest and most invigorating air, are of no avail, if the patient does not find a good home, with comfortable, well ventilated rooms, and an attentive physician. It is erroneous to rely on the climate alone, to the neglect of all other curative means; *a consumptive patient must constantly be under medical supervision*, as many changes and complications arise which require advice. In former times the laudable practice prevailed among wealthy patients travelling for the benefit of their health, of being accompanied by a physician, who constantly watched every change of their disease.

Patients sojourning at a continental sanitarium or health-station have the great advantage of finding everywhere a large number of experienced physicians, who make the treatment of pulmonary diseases a specialty.

Change of air being the most reliable remedy which could benefit consumptive persons, it should be resorted to in the very beginning of the malady. It is a great mistake to believe that favourable results can be obtained by keeping patients at home, and confined to their rooms during the unfavourable fall and winter season, deeming them sufficiently protected against the inclemency of the weather by proper heating and ventilation. *The best heated and best ventilated house is no adequate substitute for the bright sun and fresh, mild air of a southern resort.* The very air of our houses is poisonous to the patient, contaminated as it is by the dust from carpets, beds, coals, streets, &c.; and to confine him for any length of time to his room is deleterious, and a loss of valuable time.

It cannot be denied that by neglect on the part of physicians of giving timely warning to persons predisposed to consumption, or by their disregard of the first symptoms of the disease, a large number of lives are sacrificed, which perhaps could have been saved by an early change of locality. On the other hand, it is also notorious that year after year quite a number of consumptive patients are sent abroad by careless or unscrupulous practitioners, who, owing to the advanced stage of the disease, are scarcely able to endure the hardships of the voyage, and often die as soon as they reach the "promised land." Such criminal carelessness, though repeatedly denounced by medical authorities, is nevertheless of daily occurrence.

Such symptoms as excessive expectoration, hectic fever, short breathing, profuse night-sweats, diarrhœa, and general debility, forbid any change of locality as a useless, and generally even dangerous undertaking; and intelligent patients of this kind should not urge the physician to send them to a climatic resort, nor should the latter allow them to leave their homes on a hopeless trip. Cavities in the lungs, if not too large, can heal, and are no absolute contra-indications to a change of air, if the other symptoms are not alarming, and the patient not so much reduced in strength as to be unfit for outdoor exercise, which is the principal and most important part of climatic treatment.

The selection of a suitable place must be left to the physician, who alone is able to decide whether a southern station, or an Alpine region, or a sea-side resort, be a proper place for the patient. Climatology is a part of medical science, every physician being expected to possess a sufficient knowledge of it.

We intend to give some general information on climatic resorts, for the benefit of those who, while travelling on the continent, become sick, and wish to remain for a time at a climatic station, or who may be sent abroad for the sole purpose of restoring their health by a change of air and a sojourn in a warm climate.

The best time to leave the north for a southern resort is the month of October. Patients should not travel alone; and, if circumstances permit, should be accompanied by a physician. Warm woollen clothing, particularly underwear, should be worn at all times, the changes of temperature being often very sudden in southern regions, and very intensely felt by sick persons; even the change from the sunny to the shady side of the streets produces a chilly feeling. No patient should, therefore, leave the room without being provided with an overcoat or woollen wrap. A further rule is, not to hire a room unless it has a southern exposure, and is provided with a stove; for, in Northern Italy, and even in Rome and Naples, fire is required on cool days.

The room should be high and airy; and narrow,

cool streets, where sunshine is a rarity, should be just as assiduously avoided as dusty and noisy ones. The floor of the room should be covered with a carpet. If the room is found to be cool or damp, it should be immediately changed. It is also advisable to hire a room and bedroom, as it is unwholesome to remain in the same room where one sleeps, when unfavourable weather forbids outdoor exercise.

A great mistake, often made by patients, is that of hurrying with railway speed from the cool, cloudy north to the warm, sunny south. Such a rapid transition from a low to a high temperature is often very injurious. They should make it a rule to travel slowly and comfortably, and to remain for a short time at an intermediate station which has a mild climate. As such stations, the numerous little villages at the Lake of Geneva may be recommended, or Meran and Botzen in the Tyrol. By residing there a few weeks, patients become accustomed to a warm climate, and may thus without apprehension travel further southward. On the return trip they should observe the same precautions.

Many patients are unfavourably impressed by noticing that a large number of natives of southern resorts succumb to the very disease of which they expect to be cured. They should not be disheartened by this circumstance, but rather consider the difference existing between themselves and the inhabitants, who remain at home all the year round, even during the unhealthy season, while they themselves may again seek change of air upon the approach of summer, or whenever the climate no longer agrees with them. Furthermore, visitors to southern resorts generally have the means of providing for healthy, comfortable rooms, suitable clothing, &c. They enjoy all the repose and comfort which a life without labour and exertion affords, and derive the greatest possible benefit from the mild climate without being influenced by any local or social disadvantage. Thus they are infinitely better situated than the large majority of the natives, who, like those of other countries, succumb to the malady chiefly in consequence of hard labour, misery, deficient clothing, scanty food, and unwholesome, overcrowded, contaminated dwellings. The populace of Nice and Palermo—places much frequented by consumptive patients from the north—furnish their quota to the immense number of victims who year after year are sacrificed to pulmonary consumption; nevertheless there need be no hesitation in recommending these places as climatic stations to northern patients, who repair thither provided with the necessary means of procuring all possible comfort.

The first rule for invalids is to regulate their mode of living in a reasonable manner; they should always bear in mind that they have left their homes for the sole purpose of recovering their health, and not for sight-seeing or pleasure. Numerous invalids, desirous of making their stay in Italy as profitable as possible, indulge in *sight-seeing*. Picture galleries, churches, old ruins, are eagerly inspected, though the cold, damp air of these buildings is a deadly poison to every patient. All those who have travelled in Italy will coincide with the author, that more unwholesome places can scarcely be found than the celebrated churches and galleries of Rome, Naples, &c. Of course the temptation is very great, but invalids must withstand it, and shun these places, even when they feel better, and believe themselves fully restored to health. A single cold contracted at one of these unhealthy galleries, or exhaustion produced by running from one church to another, or to noted ruins, will surely cause a dangerous relapse.

To travel restlessly from one city to another, in order to satisfy a vain curiosity, is equally injurious; invalids should remember that they are not tourists, that rest and comfort are indispensable for their recovery, and that every over-fatigue and exhaustion will do incalculable harm.

The efficacy of a southern climate depends on several circumstances, which, combined, constitute what is called its salubrity. These are, a moderate warmth, equability of temperature, absence of cold and rough winds, purity and relative humidity of air, comfortable arrangements, and a large number of clear, bright days.

Sick persons, especially consumptive ones, are very sensitive in regard to cold air. They feel cheerful and at ease on mild, warm summer days; while a sudden change to cold, rough weather, often proves pernicious, their vitality being too much impaired to overcome the injurious effects of such a change. The steady, warm temperature of a southern resort is very apt to keep a patient in a comfortable condition.

Warm air acts as a sedative, and is therefore very suitable to phthisical patients. But warm air does not mean *hot* air, and patients who believe the warmest place to be the best for their lungs, are greatly mistaken; for great heat is relaxing and enervating, and the hot summer of many southern stations is not at all adapted to patients. Even in our northern climate, excessive heat breeds disease and contagion; and those whose means permit rush to cool country places in order to inhale fresh, pure air.

Equability of temperature is another necessary requirement of a proper resort, though it does not mean an absence of all currents of air, which are necessary for purifying the atmosphere. But the variations should be moderate; an imperative requisite, however, is an entire exemption from cold, chilly north winds.

A moderate *humidity* of air is considered salubrious on account of its sedative effect, and consumptives generally feel very comfortable when the air is moderately most.

A *clear sky* and a *bright sunshine* are by far the most important factors in the climatic treatment of pulmonary consumption, all the expected and desired benefit being dependent on the number of clear, sunny days, which enable the patient to inhale the warm out-door air; therefore, that winter resort is the best which offers the largest number of fine, warm days, and the most frequent opportunity for out-door exercise.

Invalids should leave the dwelling after breakfast, and remain out-doors as long as the sun shines. From 10 a.m. to 3·30 p.m. they should shun their hotels or boarding-houses, and enjoy the bright sunshine and pure air. They should take moderate exercise, which is wholesome, as it improves the appetite and strengthens the digestion; but all fatigue must be strictly avoided, consumptives being obliged to economize their strength. Those who are too feeble to promenade, may seat themselves on a warm, sunny spot, and inhale the mild air.

As *purity of air* and immunity from noxious gases and putrefactive germs is chiefly prevalent in country places, it must be conceded that the numerous small towns of Italy, particularly those in the vicinity of the Mediterranean Sea, which are much patronized as health resorts, not only enjoy that purity in a high degree, but also possess the other requisites above mentioned. However, where there is much sunshine, there is often much shade; and so it is here. Many of these places have the great disadvantage of being built upon lime soil, from which a great amount of lime dust constantly arises. Those who have made a tour along the coast of the beautiful *Riviera di ponente* will surely recollect the thick layer of dust which covered their faces and garments. However, great efforts are being made at the most popular places to remedy this evil.

The accommodations at hotels and boarding-houses are generally satisfactory, those much patronized by English being the best arranged. English and German physicians practise at nearly every southern health-station, and patients should not omit to consult one of the resident physicians immediately on their arrival, and before making further arrangements.

Among the large number of visitors who congregate at these places, patients will always meet some one with whom they can keep up a pleasant social intercourse; this is a very important point, as it prevents them from brooding over their real or fancied complaints. They should also exert themselves to find out some suitable occupation, in order to spend the time usefully, and keep the mind free from all unnecessary distressing meditations. An unhappy state of mind is always an obstacle to recovery, and idleness leads to it.

Invalids should abstain from all excitement in the shape of theatrical performances, concerts, evening parties, &c., in warm, ill-ventilated rooms, the air of which is poisoned by the exhalations of a large crowd of visitors; they should likewise abstain from the luxury of opulent *table d'hôte* dinners, and especially from the delicious cakes, tarts, and other indigestible dishes which usually form their chief attraction. Plain but substantial and well-prepared food is best suited for invalids. Those who have not the moral strength to adhere to the rules of a sound dietetic regimen and to renounce all excesses of living, should rather remain at home, and save themselves the expense and trouble of a long voyage.

All writers on climatology warn invalids from returning prematurely to the north; but their advice is rarely heeded. Most of the southern resorts already become very warm at the end of April; and patients, who generally long for their relatives and friends, cannot be convinced that their homes are still cold and uncomfortable, and expose themselves too soon to the inclemency of the northern climate. Having by their sojourn in the south become more susceptible to the change of temperature, they are in the greatest danger of taking cold, thereby losing all the benefit of their trip to the south. They should not leave the southern resorts before the end of May ; a sojourn of a few weeks at one of the intermediate stations on the Lake of Geneva, or in the Tyrol, will prove of great advantage.

Invalids who have considerably improved by the change of climate, are generally easily deluded by the apparent subsidence of most of the unfavourable symptoms, and become less cautious ; they should remember that consumption is a perfidious disease, and is often only slumbering, when they, under the impression that they are cured, neglect all necessary precautions, thereby running the risk of a speedy and fatal relapse.

In order to obtain a permanent cure, which can only be hoped for in the earliest stages of the disease, it is absolutely necessary to pass several seasons in a warm climate. If the disease is so far advanced that only a prolongation of life can be aimed at, a permanent residence in the south is the only means of procuring the desired result.

In the foregoing pages we have spoken of the southern health-stations with regard to pulmonary consumption. But there are other complaints, which are equally as much benefited by the change of climate. Of these the following may be mentioned : rheumatism, gout, all chronic affections of the throat and bronchial tubes, particularly obstinate catarrhs, which are often the forerunners of phthisis. For protracted whooping-cough a change of climate is eminently profitable, also for rickety and scrofulous children, who need constant out-door exercise.

Persons affected with neuralgia, or those slowly convalescing from exhausting diseases, also derive great benefit from a sojourn in a southern climate. Hypochondriacs, and all others who suffer from nervous depression caused by excessive mental labour or trouble, will undoubtedly be greatly benefited by a trip to the south. This is also highly recommended for old, decrepid persons, who, more than other individuals, need a warm, mild air, in order to keep up their vitality ; a protracted sojourn in the sunny south, at a resort which is provided with all necessary comfort, will aid in prolonging their lives.

We shall now briefly enumerate the most noted southern winter stations, which are recommended on account of the salubrity of climate, complete arrangements, &c.

MADEIRA, one of the Canary Islands, is one of the most favoured resorts, and especially patronized by the English. It has no winter, and a temperate summer. Patients who during the summer feel too warm at Funchal, the principal place of Madeira, need not leave the island, but may repair to other places of higher elevation, as Santa Cruz, Camacho, &c. Madeira possesses all the requirements of a first-class climatic station—a warm, equable climate in winter and summer, mild sea-air, comfortable arrangements, and experienced physicians of the principal nationalities, namely, English, French, and German. All writers on climatic resorts are enthusiastic in the praise of the climate, and unanimously recommend this island for consumptives, as superior to all other southern stations. The special advantages are, good boarding-houses, with clean, comfortable rooms, and reasonable prices; excellent water in great abundance, superior quality of meat, fish, vegetables, and fruit, especially strawberries and grapes, absence of dust, good sea baths, attentive inhabitants, and plenty of opportunity for entertainment and suitable social intercourse.

To the English, who for a long time have extensively patronized the island, patients are indebted for the great comforts which they obtain at Madeira.

CAIRO, in Egypt. The climate is mild and equable; there is a temperate season, lasting from October until March, during which time the temperature is similar to that of a summer in a northern region; the hot season, from March to September, is unfavourable to patients. Cloudy days are very rare, the sky being almost constantly clear and bright; the sun shines brilliantly, and the air is mild and balmy. No other climate admits of so much out-door exercise during the winter months. Among the natives, and the Europeans who permanently reside in Egypt, consumption is not a frequent disease, and consumptive patients from abroad generally feel better during their stay in Egypt. Cairo has comfortable hotels, parks, &c. There is also in the vicinity of Cairo a sanitarium for consumptives, established by Dr. Reil.

PALERMO, in Sicily, has a mild, equable, and moist climate, which is very well adapted to excitable patients. The mean winter temperature is 50°, with very few variations. Palermo has the mildest and most equable climate in Italy, and is very well suited to consumptive patients, from November until May being the most favourable time. There are numerous promenades and gardens, and the place is free from dust, but the want of comfortable dwellings is much complained of.

CATANIA, a fine city on the eastern coast of Italy, has a mean winter temperature of 50°, and a constantly moist air. It is becoming quite a popular resort, and many prefer it to Palermo. The new Hôtel Acireale, near Catania, has been erected for the special accommodation of invalids.

AJACCIO, on the island of Corsica, has a mean temperature of 54°, a mild, equable, and moist climate, and is well protected by high mountains against cold winds. It has a great number of fine, clear, sunshiny days, and, on account of its maritime situation, a mild winter and temperate summer. It is situated at the northernly end of a beautiful bay, and is surrounded by a long mountain range of 6000 to 9000 feet elevation; from the north and east it is completely sheltered; the warm southernly winds alone have free access.

The situation of Ajaccio is enthusiastically described by many writers, the bay being praised as one of the most magnificent on the globe, rivalling that of Naples. There is no dust, but an extremely pure air, excellent water and wine; there is little rain. Many promenades in the city and its environs afford pleasant opportunity for active exercise. Tropical plants, palm-trees, bananas, pine-apples, sugar-cane, &c., delight the eye of the stranger, and make a favourable, cheerful impression on his mind. The inhabitants are reported as civil and very obliging. Of late several new hotels have been erected, with comfortable arrangements and reasonable prices. On the whole the place seems eminently fitted for a winter resort for persons suffering from bronchial catarrh, asthma, and consumption.

On the Continent, the western part of the Gulf of Genoa, called *Riviera di ponente*, was for a long time considered the most favourable resort for consumptives. It is indeed one of the most blessed regions on earth, a little paradise, and the great reputation which it enjoys, is well deserved. Those of our readers who have visited that region, will surely recall with pleasure the lovely scenery along the whole shore, the forests of pines alternating with those of olive-trees, the well-cultivated gardens with an abundance of lemons, oranges, figs, and palms, the flourishing cities, the romantic rocks and hills crowned with the ruins of old castles and chapels.

The most popular stations on or near the *Riviera* are Hyères, Cannes, Nice, Mentone, San Remo.

HYÈRES, about one hour's drive from the sea-shore, has been highly praised by some authors; others, however, entirely deny its salubrity, as it is too much exposed to the violent *mistral*, which finds access from the north-west, and is accompanied by immense clouds of dust. There are fine promenades, a theatre, casino, and comfortable hotels.

CANNES, the most westernly place of the *Riviera*, has a beautiful situation on the bay of Napoule. Numerous comfortable villas and boarding-houses afford good accommodation to patients, especially those in the adjoining village *Le Cannet*, which is well-sheltered against the *mistral*, and free from dust. The climate is mild and equable, the mean temperature 48°. Cannes is the place where the immense quantities of odoriferous flowers are cultivated which are used for the preparation of odoriferous extracts and essences. There are many sunny, few cloudy or rainy days, and no foggy ones; the air is pure and balsamic. This city, which is much patronized by the English, has a casino, a theatre, gardens, reading-rooms, book-shops, &c. : prices are high.

NICE (*Nizza*), the largest and most popular of all European winter resorts, combines a beautiful situation, superb environs, and a mild climate, with the comforts of a large city. It has two theatres, concert, and reading-rooms, fine parks, &c. The grand promenade along the sea-shore, called the *Promenade des Anglais*, enjoys a wide reputation, though it is dusty, and without shade. By the river Paillon the city is divided into an eastern and western part, the latter being the head-quarters of the foreigners, and provided with the best hotels and boarding-houses. Numerous villas adorn the surrounding hills. The place is very well sheltered from the north and east, but from the west the *mistral* invades it. The climate is warm and moderately dry. The mean winter temperature is 46°—48°, with many variations and rapid changes; the mean fall temperature is 56°. There are about one hundred perfectly clear and bright days during the winter, and only fifty-three rainy days during the whole year. The difference of the temperature between the sunny and the shady side of the streets is very great, often ranging from 52°—76°; the evenings particularly are usually very cool. The fall abounds in rain, but the winter is mostly fine and mild, and the vegetation all around the city is luxuriant.

The climate of Nice is considered stimulating and tonic; the air is pure, but the dust often very annoying. Patients can enjoy out-door exercise nearly every day during the winter. Nevertheless the place is not very suitable for consumptives, on account of the sudden changes of temperature, the inferior quality of the water, the violent cool north-west winds, and the noisy life of a large city. For these reasons many authorities do not favour it as a winter resort for persons affected with lung diseases, while it is highly recommended for feeble persons, especially those convalescing from severe diseases, for rheumatic and gouty patients, and for the cure of bronchial catarrhs.

Patients should consult one of the resident physicians before taking apartments, as there is a marked difference of the climate in the diverse quarters of the city; they should not go out-doors early in the morning or late in the evening, and never without being provided with an overcoat or wrap. Extensive pleasure trips and a luxurious table are injurious.

MENTONE has in the short time of ten years become one of the most frequented winter resorts. It is a pretty little city, with 5000 inhabitants, situated on a charming bay, and is very well protected by high mountains against the cool north-west and east winds, only warm southern winds having free access. Near the shore, as well as on the slope of the hills away from the sea, are many good hotels, boarding-houses, and fine, comfortable villas, all affording good accommodation for invalids. The place is crowded during the winter, especially by English and French.

The climate is very mild, very equable, and moderately dry. Sudden changes from cold to warm are of very rare occurrence, the sky being constantly clear and bright; during the whole winter patients can take out-door exercise. Dews are frequent and dangerous, and the nights often cold; fogs never occur. The mean temperature is 48°—50°, and about 214 days of the year are sunny and clear. A sojourn at Mentone will prove profitable in cases of consumption, chronic bronchial and laryngeal catarrh, rheumatism, and gout; it is also highly recommended for scrofulous children. Excitable persons, or those predisposed to hemorrhage of the lungs, are not advised to reside there.

A considerable number of experienced English, German, and French physicians practise there during the winter.

SAN REMO very much resembles Mentone; it is well sheltered from the north, and tolerably well from the east and west; the climate is warm, equable, and mild, the vegetation luxuriant, and the water good. Mean winter temperature, 48°—50°; only thirty-five days during the whole season are rainy. The inhabitants are reported to be honest and well educated. There are several good hotels and boarding-houses, cafés, a casino, &c. Of late years the place has grown very much in importance, and has become quite a popular rival of Mentone and the other Italian resorts.

Rome, Naples, and *Venice* have been at all times

T

more or less patronized by invalids from northern regions.

ROME, the eternal city, the Mecca of all those who love science and art, and are desirous of seeing some relics of the grandeur of that ancient mistress of the world—is no suitable place for consumptive patients, as rapid changes of temperature, rough winds, damp air, cool nights, and narrow, cold streets, are decidedly injurious to any invalid. From the earliest times malaria has made Rome notorious, and every season some of the foreign residents are carried off by that unrelenting enemy. Even healthy persons, if not endowed with a good, strong constitution, cannot for any length of time endure the frequent variations of temperature, the cold and damp air of the numerous churches and galleries which all strangers are in the habit of visiting, and the uncomfortable, cold rooms of hotels and private houses, the arrangements for heating being very imperfect in Rome as well as in most of the southern cities.

NAPLES has also a very variable climate, sudden changes being of frequent occurrence during the winter season. This city is very noisy, and not suitable for persons requiring a quiet resort.

VENICE has been highly praised by many climatologists, while others condemn it as unfit for a climatic resort. It is exposed to the violent, cold, north-east wind, called the *Bora*, and to the hot, oppressive, south-east wind (*Scirocco*). The water is bad, and the foul odours emanating from the canals and lagunes are neither pleasant nor salubrious. Though the gondola-trips on the *Canal grande* are delightful

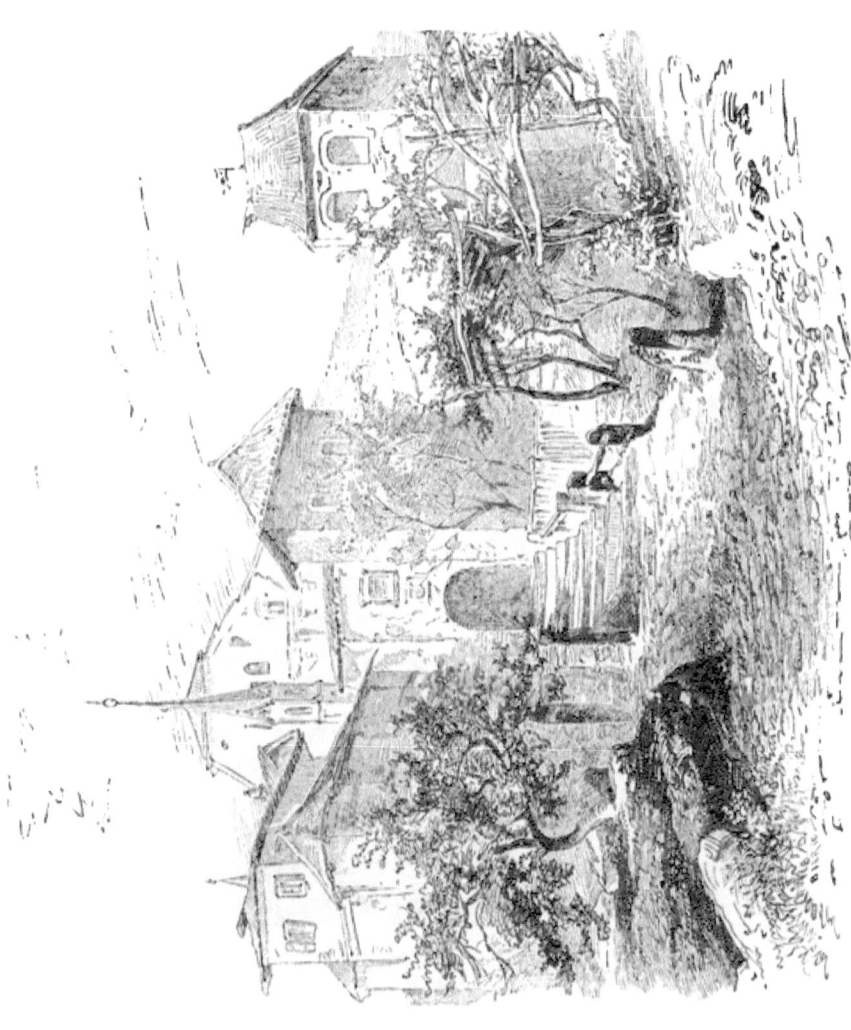

and highly interesting, they are, nevertheless, no compensation for fine promenades, the most essential requisite of a climatic resort, the want of which is a very great drawback to Venice.

Venice seems to me to be no suitable resort as a permanent residence for consumptives, but it is becoming very popular as an intermediate fall and spring station for patients going to or returning from southern resorts.

MERAN, in the Tyrol, a little city with 4000 inhabitants, and 1000 feet above the sea, is perhaps the most popular of these intermediate stations. Its situation in the charming valley of the Etsch is magnificent; fine promenades, beautiful environs, a new, handsome *Kurhaus* with café and restaurant, good hotels and villas, with comfortable arrangements, render a temporary residence at Meran very pleasant. The place is sheltered from the north and east by high mountains of 5000 to 7000 feet elevation. Meran has a vast reputation as a climatic resort, and is crowded during the fall, when the grape-cure begins. The large number of houses which seem to have been recently erected, prove the growing prosperity and popularity of this little city.

Notwithstanding a large number of fine, clear days, the winter is not very favourable to consumptive patients, as the insulation is greatly impaired by the high, snow-covered mountains. The warm rays of the sun reach the valley only from eleven to three o'clock, and at times it is very cold indeed. The mean temperature of January is only 31°, of February 40°, of March 56°.

A sojourn at Meran is highly beneficial for scrofulous children, decrepid old persons, over-worked business men, and delicate, anæmic ladies.

BOTZEN, and the neighbouring village GRIES, about three hours distant from Meran, are also recommended as climatic stations.

ARCO, a little city with 2700 inhabitants, beautifully situated in the southern Tyrol, near the *Lago di Garda*, has in December and January a higher temperature than Meran. It is eminently fit for an intermediate station, and the number of visitors is steadily increasing. An elegant, spacious *Kurhaus*, with a large concert *salon*, billiard, reading, and sitting-rooms, and sixty high and airy rooms for the accommodation of patients, was erected in 1878. A large number of villas, surrounded by fine gardens, afford pleasant accommodations to visitors.

MONTREUX, VEVEY, CLARENS, and other places on the eastern shore of the Lake of Geneva, are also suitable stations for invalids returning from the south.

The cure of consumption by a prolonged residence in *elevated regions*, aided by proper medical treatment, has, for almost two decades, attracted the attention of physicians and the public in general. The pioneer of this movement was Dr. Brehmer of *Görbersdorf* (Silesia), who opened the *first sanitarium* on an elevated point, and introduced the cold water cure into the treatment of consumption. His establishment and method of treatment at present enjoy a great reputation, and the opposition to his method on the part of the regular practitioners, is gradually subsiding.

Though the establishment is a little out of the regular route of tourists, physicians should not on this account permit themselves to be deterred from visiting it and examining the arrangements; they will be highly satisfied, and no matter what their views of the method of treatment may be, they will surely coincide with the author in the opinion that the establishment fully deserves the high reputation which it has already obtained.

There was once a general prejudice among the members of the profession against the climatic treatment of phthisis on elevated regions, especially when continued during the winter, and a far greater one still against the treatment by cold water. It would annoy the reader to enter into a long discourse on the *rationale* of this method, but the fact cannot be denied, that beneficial results have been obtained at the sanitariums of Görbersdorf, Davos, &c., though it will take a long time yet before this question can be satisfactorily settled.

To send patients to high altitudes for a stay during the summer, has been a favourite remedy from the earliest times; and many places of the kind in all parts of the globe are crowded with consumptives. However, it was quite a new feature to furnish a sanitarium with all the necessary comfort, and put it under the management of experienced physicians, who devote their time to the special treatment of consumption, and to keep patients in a place so provided during the winter months. A wilderness, however beautiful and healthful the climate may be, and however high it may be situated above the sea, is no suitable abode for patients who require perfect arrangements in regard to lodgings and food, and constant medical supervision. Sanitariums in elevated regions, which answer all requirements, for the present exist only on the continent, and are becoming very popular. Görbersdorf and Davos are patronized by patients of all nationalities, who remain there during the winter.

The principal requirements for a sanitarium are, a high situation, sufficient protection against rough winds, and fresh, pure air. Sanitariums on high regions have a great advantage over their competitors, the southern resorts, in point of fresh, invigorating air, absence of dust and germs, perfect quiet, &c.

The sanitarium at Görbersdorf is a very extensive and complete establishment, and fully deserves our commendation. Few persons know how to appreciate the skill, knowledge, and administrative capacity which are required in order to establish and arrange a large complete medical institution, and the difficulties of managing it in so perfect a manner as is done at Görbersdorf.

The sanitarium is situated in a small valley of the Silesian mountains, 1900 feet above the sea, pretty well sheltered by mountains of 3000 feet elevation. The air is fresh and bracing, and very rich in ozone, the water is pure and refreshing. There is a spacious *Kurhaus*—a grand building in purely Gothic style, 500 feet long, containing large dining-rooms, a winter garden, and a large concert-hall in Gothic style. There are also 110 high, airy, comfortable rooms for the accommodation of patients, neatly furnished, and exceedingly clean; each room is provided with an hygrometer to control the humidity of the air, and with excellent ventilation. The whole building is heated by hot water. Three villa houses are close by the *Kurhaus*, with accommodations for fifty-three patients. There are also eighteen houses in the village, with 250 rooms, where patients are received. A separate building for the application of cold water is situated in the pine forest, a few hundred feet distant from the *Kurhaus*. Opposite to the latter is the great dairy-farm, with a large number of excellent cows and goats, which furnish the immense quantities of milk required for the patients.

In front of the *Kurhaus* a fine garden is laid out, stocked with domestic and exotic plants; and adjoining it are the promenades, the most important part of this and every other properly-arranged sanitarium. The arrangement of these promenades bears testimony to the intelligence and skill of the leading spirit of the establishment, everything being carefully adjusted with respect to the wants of the invalids; covering an area of about eighty acres, the shady walks gradually and smoothly lead up to the highest elevation. On well-selected spots more than 300 benches are placed, affording shady resting-places to the invalids when ascending the hills. All these walks are through pine-woods, which fill the air with a balsamic odour. A large number of hammocks are suspended among the pine-trees, affording on warm days a pleasant opportunity for an afternoon siesta. In short, everything is done for the purpose of enticing the patients to spend their whole time in the open air. The gist of the whole treatment consists in the enjoyment of proper food and pure air, under the strictest surveillance of physicians, everything being controlled by Dr. Brehmer and three assistants. Every patient is carefully examined and observed, and a diary is kept of each respective case. The application of the cold water takes place under their personal supervision, and is entirely omitted as soon as contra-indications arise ; as, for instance, a want of reactive power, hemorrhage, &c. Dr. Brehmer is by no means a fanatic in his advocacy of the cold-water treatment, but applies it with discretion, and at all events deserves credit for the courage and energy he exhibited by introducing into the treatment of consumption such a heroic method, which is in absolute contrast to the doctrines of the old medical school.

Eating, drinking, and promenading being almost the only business of the day, special attention is paid to the bill of fare, which presents a fine array of substantial, nourishing dishes, of the best quality. Five times a day the bell calls the boarders to the dining-rooms : for breakfast (seven to eight), lunch (ten to eleven), dinner (half-past twelve), coffee (four to five), supper (six to seven). Excellent meat and bread, large quantities of pure milk, good Hungarian wine, and fresh vegetables, are the medicines applied by the physicians of the place. At ten o'clock p.m. all patients retire.

By the constant supervision on the part of the physicians, patients are kept back from all those excesses in which consumptive patients so often indulge, thereby inflicting upon themselves irreparable harm.

Patients should never expect to be cured by a short

stay at a sanitarium; it has already been stated that a diseased lung can be cured, if proper remedies are applied in the early stages of the affliction; but it requires months, and even years, to perfect a cure, and a too hasty departure often frustrates the good results already obtained. *Patience and perseverance* should be the parole of all invalids, and especially of all consumptives.

If the author should perhaps have devoted too much time and space to the description of that model sanitarium at Görbersdorf, he hopes to be excused by the importance of the subject, which is a vital question for thousands of unfortunate patients, who long for help, no matter what may be the expense or trouble.

At Görbersdorf another sanitarium has recently been opened, which, however, bears no comparison with that of Dr. Brehmer.

DAVOS, in Switzerland, also enjoys an immense reputation for the cure of consumptives. It has an elevation of 5000 feet above the sea, and the treatment is shaped after Dr. Brehmer's method. The place is well sheltered from the north; even in the winter the heat at noon is often intense, but the nights are almost too cool. However, it is a first-class winter resort, of great repute, and extensively patronized, has comfortable boarding-houses with excellent table, and good arrangements for cold-water treatment. There are also experienced physicians, who make the treatment of consumption their special study. Feverish patients, and those possessing little power of reaction, are not advised to go to Davos. The time when the snow melts, viz., from March to

June, is considered particularly unfavourable at this place.

AUSSEE, which has already been mentioned as an excellent brine bath, has attained a reputation as a climatic health resort through the sanitarium of Dr. Schreiber. The establishment is pretty well arranged, but changed hands several years ago; and as it is no more carried on under the special supervision of a physician, it can hardly be considered a sanitarium. On my last visit to the place, in August, 1879, I was reliably informed that Dr. Schreiber within a short time intends to establish another sanitarium, on a grand scale, on one of the highest spots in Aussee, which affords a beautiful view of the charming village and the romantic lake. Aussee is surely a magnificent place for a sanitarium, having an elevation of 2000 feet, and a fresh, bracing Alpine air.

Beside these regular sanitariums, there are hundreds of places in all the mountain regions of Central Europe which are praised as resorts for invalids. Being mostly intended for the reception of summer visitors, they are called summer stations, or *Sommerfrischen*, the latter expression being very popular among the Germans. To persons whose nervous system is deranged in consequence of excessive mental labour, or to convalescents after acute diseases, or to others exhausted by chronic affections, a stay of several months at one of these resorts will be exceedingly beneficial. The practice of visiting such places is becoming more popular every year, and many may consider it a peculiar habit of modern times. But at all ages summer resorts have existed and been patronized, and those of the Romans were notorious for elegance, luxury, and extravagance. But there is a great difference between ancient and modern times, inasmuch as nowadays, through the facilities afforded by railways and steamboats, persons of moderate means are enabled to enjoy the benefit of a summer resort, whilst previous to the general introduction of steam, only the *upper ten* had this privilege. This laudable and beneficial luxury is at present indulged in to such an extent, that in the spring of every year a regular hægira takes place from the overcrowded cities to the elevated regions.

It would be impossible to enumerate all the summer resorts, as there is hardly a single spot in the mountains which is not advertised as a beautiful, very healthy *Sommerfrische*, with unsurpassed accommodations. To English and Americans travelling near the Rhine, the little mountain villages of the Black Forest, the Bavarian Alps, and Switzerland, may be recommended; to those residing at Dresden and Berlin, those of the Saxon, Swiss, and the Riesengebirge. In Austria—the Tyrol, Styria, and Salzburg have an abundance of pleasant and healthy summer stations. But it seems proper to repeat, that consumptive patients should resort to a regular sanitarium, where they are sure of receiving good medical attendance.

A few words remain to be said of the sea-side resorts on the Continent. Many patients, after having finished a course of treatment at Karlsbad, Marienbad, or some other spa, are advised to take sea baths, in order to regain their bodily strength; others are sent thither for the only purpose of inhaling the fresh, bracing sea-air. Sea baths are an excellent remedy for persons with a tender skin, who are inclined to catch cold at every change of temperature. They are also of great benefit in chronic-bronchial catarrhs, scrofula, neuralgia of the head (hemicrania), general debility, &c. There are several excellent sea baths on the coast of the German Ocean (North Sea). We mention the following as the most popular :—

OSTEND, on the Belgian coast, the most celebrated sea bath on the Continent, patronized by visitors from all parts of Europe, but too noisy for those who are fond of quiet living. All the arrangements are first class, and the prices high. The place has an excellent beach, and strong waves.

SCHEVENINGEN, on the Dutch coast, near the Hague, is a fashionable bath, with perfect arrangements, and high prices.

There are four other sea baths, on four islands near the German coast, which are extensively patronized by the better class of Germans. These islands are: Sylt, Norderney, Borkum, Heligoland (the last-named belonging to the British Government); they are not frequented by English or Americans, though they ought to be patronized on account of the good sea bathing, complete arrangements, and moderate prices.

SYLT, near the Sleswig coast, has superb waves and a very strong, bracing air; it is, perhaps, the most forcible sea bath on the German Ocean. But the accommodations are not so perfect as they should be, the inhabitants being somewhat phlegmatic, and slow to improve.

NORDERNEY has very good arrangements, an excellent beach, and good waves. Bath life is very pleasant and everything is done for the comfort of the visitors. The place is crowded in the height of the season.

BORKUM, west of Norderney, is also becoming quite popular, great efforts being made to satisfy the visitors.

HELIGOLAND is the most fashionable of these four places. It has comfortable arrangements, a bracing sea-air, and excellent surf-bathing. The place where the patients bathe is situated on a dune, formerly connected with the island, but now separated from it, and bathers are obliged to cross in a boat, which is somewhat inconvenient.

CHAPTER II.

MISCELLANEOUS CURES.

BESIDES the numerous mineral springs and health resorts, the armamentory of the Continental practitioners is stocked with a large number of other weapons, which they skilfully handle in the combat with disease. Peat, mud, sand, tan, malt, pine-needle, herb baths; grapes, milk, whey, koumis, herb-bitters, cold water in every shape, and many other substances of the organic and inorganic kingdoms, are summoned in order to combat, and if possible to vanquish, the common enemy.

Foreigners visiting the German watering places will notice with surprise an immense number of advertisements, either in newspapers or in the shape of pamphlets, or placards, &c., extolling one or the other of these remedies. The following brief notes will give all information that is required in order to appreciate the real virtue of those which at present still enjoy a great popularity. In these things, as in so many others, fashion reigns with despotic power, and remedies which a short time ago seemed to have the firmest hold in the estimation of the profession, are now deposed without mercy.

Peat and mud baths are at present perhaps the most favoured remedies on the Continent, there being scarcely any watering place, at least of those enumerated in this treatise, without these appliances. But they are no specialty of modern medical science, as, according to the reports of Pliny, Galen, and others, even the old Romans were in the habit of using them. There is no essential difference in regard to the physiological action and therapeutical application between peat and mud baths, though their chemical composition is not identical.

Peat baths are made of the peat or moor earth, of which immense deposits are found in all parts of the globe. The peat having been powdered and sifted, is mixed with mineral water or plain hot water, until it has attained the consistency of a well-prepared poultice. Such a preparation presents the appearance of a thick, black, pappy substance, not very alluring indeed, as it resembles far more a heap of that ugly mud which street sweepers often collect in the streets than an important medical appliance, and to jump into that unsightly mass seems to require a good deal of courage. A patient who takes a peat bath at first feels a little excited, and oppressed by the heavy weight of the peat; but this feeling rapidly passes off, and soon he is perfectly at ease. The only trouble he has is in obtaining a firm hold; for as the pappy liquid has a higher specific gravity than the human body, he is lifted, and experiences some difficulty in lying or sitting in the bath.

Peat is produced by decomposition of organic substances, and consists of humic acid, resin, silicic acid, a large quantity of vegetable remains, sulphate of iron, magnesia, &c.; it also contains sulphuretted hydrogen, carbonic acid, and nitrogen. The temperature of the peat bath is higher than that of the mineral water bath, namely 100° and even more.

Peat baths produce irritation of the skin, which is manifested by redness and increased perspiration, and sometimes even by eruptions; they have a calming effect on the cutaneous nerves, and are strong resolvents for all kinds of exudations. They are very efficacious in rheumatic and gouty exudations, and thickening of the joints; paralytic and hysterical patients are also much benefited; in neuralgia, especially sciatica, great success is claimed for the treatment by peat baths.

The duration of a peat bath varies from fifteen to forty-five minutes. There is always in the bathing-room another bathing tub, filled with warm water, which the patient uses after leaving the peat bath; but he should not remain therein any longer than necessary for cleaning the skin.

Mud baths are employed for the same diseases as peat baths, and their efficacy in chronic diseases of the skin is particularly praised. Mud is a deposit from mineral waters, especially from sulphur springs, and contains the chemical constituents and some organic substances which are usually found in these.

Sand baths. In tropical climates the sand as heated by the sun is used for arenation. On the Continent, sand is artificially heated on sheets of iron. In order to prepare the sand bath, the bottom of the bathing-tub is covered with the hot sand to the height of five inches; the patient lies down on it, and is then covered with five inches of sand, which has a temperature of 116°—122°. Having remained therein from forty-five to sixty minutes, he takes a warm water bath, for the purpose of washing off the sand, of which a considerable quantity usually adheres to the skin. The sand bath produces a profuse perspiration, whereby one, and even two pounds of fluid, are excreted.

Sand baths were extensively applied by the Roman and Arabian physicians; they are of great advantage in chronic rheumatism, and in exudations in and around the joints resulting therefrom; they are also recommended in paralysis caused by suppressed perspiration.

Pine-needle baths are likewise very extensively used in Germany. A fluid extract, of greenish colour and aromatic odour, is prepared from the fresh leaves of pine trees; about two ounces of it, mixed with the necessary quantity of warm water, are sufficient for a bath. A decoction. freshly prepared every day, is also used, six, ten, or fifteen quarts being added to a bath. The temperature varies from 92°—108°, according to the nature of the disease and the constitution of the patient. These baths, which fill the whole bathing-room with an aromatic and very agreeable odour, strongly stimulate the skin and the cutaneous nerves. Chronic rheumatism of the muscles and joints is particularly benefited by them; on account of their invigorating action, they are very suitable for such feeble, enervated patients as are unable to undergo an energetic treatment by warm mineral springs. They are also recommended in neuralgic affections.

Herb baths were for centuries in great favour with the physicians, but for the present they are out of fashion. Decoctions of a large number of aromatic plants, as peppermint, thyme, fennel, cummin, marjoram, rosemary, lavender, calmus, and many others, were used for the preparation of these baths, which were administered to enervated persons, especially to weak children.

Milk and whey cures play an important *rôle* at the Continental watering places, there being scarcely any spa which does not advertise "that excellent whey, prepared by a genuine Swiss from Appenzell, is at hand."

Milk of cows, goats, ewes, asses, and mares is used as nutriment, and for the treatment of various diseases. Milk contains water, fat (butter), casein, sugar, and some salts, in the following proportion :—

	Cow.	Goat.	Ewe.	Asses.	Mares.
Water	85·705	86·358	83·989	91·029	82·837
Solid constituents	14·295	13·642	16·011	8·976	17·163
Casein	4·828	3·360	5·342	2·018	1·641
Albumen	0·576	1·299	—	—	—
Butter	4·305	4·357	5·890	1·256	6·872
Milk-sugar	4·307	4·004	4·098	5·702	8·650
Salts	0·549	0·622	0·681	—	—

The salts are chloride of potass, chloride of sodium, phospate of lime, and magnesia.

The composition of milk varies with the species of the animal which yields it, the food upon which it is fed, and the region in which it is reared. Our table shows the mare's milk as containing the largest amount of mineral constituents; it has the largest quantity of sugar and butter, but the smallest amount of casein. Asses' milk is the poorest in solid constituents and butter; cows' and ewes' milk is the richest in casein.

When milk is coagulated, the casein and butter are separated from the serum, which remains fluid, and contains salts and milk-sugar, and is called *whey*. Mares' milk brought to fermentation is called *kumys*, which is the favourite beverage of the Bashkirs and Kirghis, the nomads of the great Russian steppes.

The milk we drink is coagulated by the gastric juice, but is soon again dissolved and digested. No other animal or vegetable nutriment is so rapidly, readily, and completely digested and absorbed, as milk. Nevertheless, there are many persons who do not well bear it, and feel a pressure in the epigastric region when commencing a milk cure. Milk favours the accumulation of fat; it is therefore the practice of the little African potentates to force their wives to drink daily several quarts of milk, in order to fatten them, the fattest being considered the most beautiful. Kumys has likewise a fattening tendency.

It is reported that Hippocrates, the father of medical science, employed large quantities of milk as a remedial agent. In the treatment of consumption, ulceration of the stomach, &c., milk has always been considered an important auxiliary. Even whey was already employed by the ancient physicians.

Milk treatment is very much recommended in all affections of the larynx and lungs, especially in all stages of pulmonary consumption. Splendid results are often obtained by the exclusive use of a milk diet in chronic ulcerations of the stomach. Patients take the milk warm as drawn from the cow; but there is no harm in boiling it, for those who prefer it so. From two to six ounces three or four times a day are sufficient in the beginning, the quantity being gradually increased. If patients tire of it, or do not well bear it, the quantity should be reduced. At first nothing is taken besides the milk but some white bread; after a while more substantial food is allowed.

Whey-cures are far more popular than milk-cures, though at present they are not so extensively applied as during the first half of the present century. Whey is prepared by adding a piece of a calf's stomach to boiling milk, whereby coagulation is procured. An analysis made by Dr. Valentiner shows the following composition of different kinds of whey.

One thousand parts of whey contain :—

	Cow.	Goat.	Ewe.
Water	932·6	933·8	919·6
Albuminates	10·8	11·4	21·3
Milk-sugar	51·3	45·3	50·7
Fat	1·2	3·7	2·5
Salts	4·1	5·8	5·9

There is no great difference in the therapeutical action, whether a patient take cow, or goat, or ewe whey. It has been contended that goat whey has a special beneficial action on consumptive patients, and cow whey on those affected with diseases of the abdominal organs, while ewe whey was considered the most nourishing of the three; but we have no proof of such an assertion.

The friends of the whey treatment seem to base its therapeutical value upon the nourishing action of the whey; but many practitioners think very little of it, and prefer pure milk as a far more efficacious and nourishing drink, though it cannot be denied that whey is often well borne and digested in cases where milk causes indigestion.

Whey increases the secretions of the intestinal canal, the kidneys, and the skin, and promotes the change of tissue; it also acts as a mild aperient.

In cases of incipient phthisis, whey is highly recommended by many practitioners, particularly where there is an irritation of the bronchial tubes, its action being that of a mild anti-catarrhal remedy. In chronic catarrh of the larynx and the bronchial tubes, whey alleviates the troublesome cough and facilitates the expectoration. These are the cases which derive the most benefit from a whey-cure. The curative effects of whey are also much praised in hemorrhoids and retarded circulation in the abdominal organs, the so-called *plethora abdominalis* of the German physicians.

Whey should be taken with great caution by patients who are predisposed to congestions of the lungs and hemorrhage, or by those who suffer from catarrh of the stomach. It should not be applied in the advanced stages of consumption.

The best time for a whey-cure is the summer. The temperature of this pleasant beverage is 105° or more; the smallest quantity which is taken per day is half a quart, the largest about two quarts. Patients mus promenade while drinking, in order to promote its digestion. They should not take breakfast too soon after having swallowed the last portion of the prescribed quantity, and should strictly abstain from all indigestible food.

Whey-cures are often combined with mineral water cures; alkaline waters in particular are very often mixed with warm whey, and their efficacy is said to be considerably promoted by this method.

Kumys contains water, alcohol, carbonic acid, and that portion of the sugar which has not fermented. It is exceedingly nourishing, the nomads of the Russian steppes living almost solely on this nutriment during the whole summer. It is a pleasant, acidulous, cooling drink, quenching thirst and hunger, and can be taken in large quantities without disturbing the digestion. The effect of a kumys diet is an increase of appetite and weight; weak and emaciated persons soon become strong and fat.

Of late years kumys has obtained a very great reputation as a curative agent in consumption. The fact that this disease is unknown among the nomads of the steppes led to the supposition that kumys was the cause of that immunity; but we would rather suggest that the fresh, pure air of the steppes is the real cause of that healthy state. Nevertheless, enough cases are reported by experienced practitioners to prove the efficacy of kumys in incipient consumption; the hectic fever decreases during its administration, the cough and expectoration are alleviated and gradually cease, the weight increases, the emaciated body fattens, and night-sweats disappear.

In order to enable patients to drink kumys without being obliged to travel to the steppes, and live like nomades, several establishments for the preparation of kumys have been erected in Germany, as for instance at Wiesbaden, Bremerhafen, &c. The diet during the kumys cure consists of mutton and bread.

Grape cures are also much favoured by German physicians. Grapes are very rich in sugar and various salts, and on the absorption of these substances the efficacy of the grape cure depends. Their chemical composition varies considerably, according to the soil where they are cultivated, the manner of cultivation, and the greater or lesser heat of the particular season. In warm climates the grape juice contains more sugar than in cold ones; hot seasons yield a sweeter wine than cold ones.

The principal constituents of the grape-juice are tartrates of lime and potass, chloride of sodium, silicates, phosphates, albumen, mucose, sugar, and water. The proportion of the sugar is $2\frac{1}{2}$ to 5 ounces in 16 ounces grape juice (Braun).

Grape-juice increases the secretion of the saliva, augments the appetite, and stimulates the action of the bowels. A patient who has consumed a moderate quantity of grapes has a feeling of fulness in the epigastric region; frequent eructation soon occurs, caused by carbonic acid which forms in the stomach. The pulse becomes fuller and accelerated, and the head dizzy; palpitation of the heart is sometimes noticed; and hemorrhage from the nose, and even from the lungs may be produced. Perspiration and secretion of urine increase, the secretion of the mucous membrane of the intestinal canal is greatly stimulated, and frequent fluid evacuations take place. These symptoms pass off as soon as the system is accustomed to the grape diet; the appetite improves, the evacuations become regular and less watery, and the change of tissue is considerably promoted.

Grapes seem to favour the accumulation of fat, and emaciated persons have often been observed to become fatter by the grape diet. But it is also contended that the fresh air and the increased appetite, which cause the patients to consume immense quantities of food during the grape cure, are more apt to produce that fattening effect than the grape juice.

However, there are many practitioners who consider the grape juice a curative agent of great virtue in consumptive cases on account of its nourishing property. Sugar having always been considered a valuable remedy in phthisis, we should infer that grape juice, which is so rich in grape sugar, would also act very beneficially, and trustworthy physicians give good accounts of the results achieved by grape treatment in the early stages of the disease.

Grape diet has proved an excellent remedy in enlargement of the liver; it is also of great advantage in cases of congestions of the brain produced by excessive mental labour or excitement. As mild aperients, grapes are often employed for habitual constipation and hemorrhoids. The grape treatment is also highly recommended for chronic catarrh of the respiratory and digestive organs.

The time for grape cures is the fall, from the middle of September until the end of October. The grapes must be ripe, but patients should not swallow the skin; nor should they go to the vineyards in the morning in order to eat the fresh grapes, as many are in the habit of doing, as there is always great danger of catching cold. They should eat one and a half or two pounds of grapes in the morning before breakfast, and one or two rolls. Two or three hours later another quantity of two or three pounds is taken, together with some white bread. About three or four hours after dinner, one and a half or two pounds are again consumed. Patients must avoid all indigestible food, especially pork, cheese, pies and cakes, salads, &c.; milk should not be drunk before or shortly after taking the grapes. Frequent active exercise is absolutely necessary, though every fatigue should be avoided. If the grapes are not tolerated by an empty stomach, patients may take a cup of tea or coffee without milk a short time before taking the first portion of the grapes. Medicines or mineral waters should not be taken during the grape cure, or shortly afterward, and a proper dietetic regimen must be kept on for several weeks after the treatment has been finished.

Fresh grape juice, squeezed out of the grapes, is used sometimes to avoid the trouble of masticating, but such practice is not commendable, as mastication is necessary for the secretion of saliva, which is considered essential for a good digestion.

The duration of a grape-treatment is usually from four to six weeks. There are some places which enjoy a great reputation as resorts for grape cures on account of the superior quality of the grapes; we mention as the most popular: *Dürkheim*, in Rhenish Bavaria; *Meran*, in the Tyrol; *Montreux*, on the lake of Geneva.

Herb-juices (*Kräutersäfte*).—At several watering places the juices obtained by squeezing fresh aromatic herbs are applied as curative agents in dispeptic cases. Numerous herbs are used for that purpose, especially those growing on Alpine heights, a specific curative power being attributed to these juices by popular belief—or rather, credulity. Such "mountain-bitters" are sold in nearly all mountain regions of Central Europe, and some places are known as specific *Kräutersaft-stations*; as, for instance, *Hall* (near Steyer), *Le Prese*, *Rheinfelden* (Switzerland), and *Goslar* (Germany), where the celebrated shoemaker, Lampe, once performed miracles by his decoctions. The *bitters* of Reichenhall and Kreuth have acquired a great popularity among the visitors of these regions.

All such preparations have no special curative effect; but as many patients believe in them, and no harm can ensue from their use, they may take them to their heart's content: *haluant sibi !*

We deem it proper to mention, for the benefit of those who are fond of *cold water treatment*, the name and location of some hydropathic institutes. There is a very large number of such establishments in Central Europe, hydropathic treatment being still very popular. But the old rigid method of the genial peasant Priessnitz is nowadays practised only in a few establishments, as a more rational method has been adopted, and most of the institutes are under the management of regular physicians.

Cold water treatment is of decided benefit in hypochondriasis, hysteria, general derangement of the nervous system, and in atony of the skin, which is the chief cause of the liability to catch cold. It has also been found useful in cases of paralysis, syphilis, anæmia, and in affections of the digestive organs.

The hydropathic institutes are generally situated in pleasant, romantic regions; such a location, a well regulated dietetic regimen, and social intercourse with the better class of society, which usually congregates at these resorts, contribute a great deal to the splendid results which are undoubtedly achieved by the cold water treatment.

We shall enumerate several establishments, which are easily accessible to English and Americans travelling on the Continent.

For the benefit of those sojourning near the Rhine or in Switzerland the following places may be mentioned:—

DIETENMÜHLE, near Wiesbaden.
NEROTHAL, near Wiesbaden.
GODESBERG, on the Rhine.
MARIENBERG, near Boppard.
MÜHLBAD, near Boppard.
BRESTENBERG, Canton Aargau,
ALBISBRUNN, Canton Zürich, } Switzerland.
SCHÖNBRUNN, near Zug,
SCHÖNEGG, on the Lake of Lucerne,

Patients residing in Dresden or Berlin may resort to—

SCHWEIZERMÜHLE near Pirna,

KÖNIGSBRUNN, near Königstein,

in Saxony, both places being picturesquely situated and well managed; prices reasonable.

Of the Austrian establishments we mention—

GRAEFENBERG, in Austrian Silesia, the mother-establishment, where Priessnitz started the cold water treatment.

KALTENLEUTGEBEN, near Vienna.

PRIESSNITZTHAL, near Vienna.

EGGENBERG, near Gratz (Styria).

OBERINAIS, near Meran (Tyrol).

CHAPTER III.

THERAPEUTICAL RECAPITULATION.

A BRIEF review of the different diseases mentioned in connexion with the therapeutical application of the various springs will, I believe, enable the reader to form a more correct opinion of their relative efficacy in each particular case; for a considerable number of mineral waters have been enumerated as equally efficient in the same disease, and the puzzled reader may desire to have a clearer idea in this respect. The best means to attain this end, will be a brief recapitulation, in which shall be indicated the various diseases treated at the springs, and the especial advantages of the various resorts with reference to particular diseases.

1. DISEASES OF THE DIGESTIVE ORGANS.

There is nothing in the world which is more frequently sinned against than the observation of a rational dietetic regimen. As a consequence the diseases of the digestive organs are far more frequent than those of the other organs, and patients seeking to restore the impaired energy of the former, throng the watering places by thousands. However, the misfortune of this class of patients is a very great one indeed ; because scarcely are they restored to health, or at least improved, when, unable to withstand the temptations of a greedy stomach, they relapse into their former habits, and the complaint soon returns. This is the reason why, year after year, so considerable a number of the same individuals are seen at the same spas, who are obliged to visit them again and again as long as they live. There are many patients who for twenty and thirty years every spring faithfully start on their yearly pilgrimage to Karlsbad and similar spas.

Dyspepsia, and catarrh of the stomach.—Dyspepsia mostly depends upon a catarrh of the stomach, but the former term is generally applied to a mild form, while the latter indicates a more inveterated or chronic condition. The catarrh is often associated with vomiting of a sour, slimy, substance, and emaciation. Alkaline and salt springs are indicated for the cure of these affections. If atony of the stomach exists, the salt springs of Kissingen, Homburg, &c., are suitable ; by stimulating the peristaltic action of the stomach, they promote the evacuation of its contents ; the application of the saline baths is a valuable auxiliary to the internal use of the salt springs. Where there is an excess of acidity, the alkaline waters, especially the alkaline-muriated springs of Ems and Gleichenberg, are of great advantage. In severe cases of chronic catarrh, which are generally complicated with constipation, the alkaline-saline (Glauber-salt) waters are the best remedies, as they gently promote the peristaltic action of the bowels. The saline waters (Kissingen, &c.) do not produce this purgative action, except by excessive doses, which easily cause irritation of the stomach and an increase of the catarrh. When great irritation and neuralgic pains are present, the warm Glaubersalt springs of Karlsbad should be resorted to, the cold Glaubersalt waters (Marienbad, Tarasp, &c.) being highly beneficial when great atony of the digestive organs complicates the case. If enlargement of the liver is combined with the catarrh, the Glaubersalt waters are the best remedies. Weak and anæmic patients use the chalybeate-saline waters of Franzensbad and Elster with great profit, or the combined salt and iron waters of Homburg.

Chronic ulcers of the stomach are effectually treated by the Karlsbad springs.

Chronic catarrh of the intestinal canal, of which diarrhœa alternating with costiveness is the principal symptom, is cured by the warm alkaline, the saline, and the earthy waters. Severe cases, particularly when combined with plethora and obesity, are most benefited by Karlsbad.

Hemorrhoids and constipation are successfully treated at Kissingen, Karlsbad, Marienbad, Tarasp, &c. The saline waters of Kissingen, Homburg, &c. are indicated when the general assimilation and nutrition are much impaired, and also when there is much nervous irritation ; Karlsbad, Marienbad, Tarasp, render excellent service to persons of great obesity, and predisposed to congestions of the internal organs.

Enlarged liver and fatty liver are cured by both the saline (Kissingen, Homburg, &c.) and the

Glaubersalt waters (Karlsbad, Marienbad, Tarasp), the latter being far more effective. The saline waters are preferred in cases of impaired nutrition; the Glaubersalt springs are unsurpassed when considerable enlargement is combined with obesity, costiveness, and a disposition to congestions.

Gall stones are cured by the thermal springs of Karlsbad, which increase the secretion of the bile, facilitate the passage and evacuation of the stones, and prevent the formation of new concretions—probably by augmenting the quantity of the soda of the bile. Tarasp is also highly recommended.

Jaundice and catarrh of the gall-ducts are also cured by the alkaline-saline waters of Karlsbad, Marienbad, &c.

Enlargement of the spleen after intermittent fever is successfully treated by saline or Glaubersalt waters. When the nutrition is much impaired and dropsy has set in, the chalybeate-saline waters of Elster or Franzensbad are indicated; peat baths are also a valuable auxiliary. The treatment should be concluded by the use of the strong iron waters of Pyrmont, Driburg, Schwalbach, &c.

2. Diseases of the Respiratory Organs.

Chronic catarrh of the throat and larynx are benefited by the alkaline waters of Salzbrunn and Neuenahr, or by the alkaline muriated waters of Ems and Gleichenberg; and if there is a scrofulous complication, by the saline waters.

Chronic bronchial catarrh and incipient phthisis.—

Salzbrunn, Ems, Gleichenberg, and Neuenahr afford great benefit for the mild forms of the catarrh and the early stages of consumption. When these affections are combined with dyspepsia and sluggishness of the bowels, the saline waters (especially Soden), which improve the nutrition, are recommended. Inhalations of atomized saline waters aid considerably. Catarrhs which are complicated with hemorrhoids and enlarged liver, derive great benefit from the use of the sulphur waters (Weilbach). Very weak patients of this kind may resort to Reinez, Cudowa, Elster, or Franzensbad.

The troublesome *dry catarrh*, which is often combined with asthma, is very much benefited by a summer sojourn in an Alpine region (Reichenhall, Kreuth, &c.), and the use of whey mixed with an alkaline muriated water, or by resorting to a southern climatic station for the winter season, the treatment being much aided by the inhalation of compressed air and atomized medicines.

Grape cures are also of great advantage in bronchial catarrh; they are recommended as so-called "after-cures," as accessories to the treatment by mineral waters.

3. Diseases of the Urinary System.

Chronic catarrh of the bladder.—Carbonate of soda being the most effectual remedy for catarrhs, it is obvious that alkaline waters, which are rich in it, will be used with great benefit in catarrh of the bladder, and great results are indeed obtained at Neuenahr,

Salzbrunn, and the other alkaline spas, if no other serious complications aggravate the case. Inveterate cases, with great atony of the bladder and impaired nutrition, are most successfully treated by the earthy waters of Wildungen. If the catarrh is associated with costiveness or retarded circulation in the abdominal organs, the waters of Karlsbad should be used.

Gravel is treated by the alkaline waters of Ems, Neuenahr, or Karlsbad, if a great irritation of the urinary system prevails. If this complication is not present, the Wildungen springs will be of great benefit. During the employment of these waters immense quantities of stones are frequently eliminated without pain.

Bright's disease of the kidneys.—The advanced stages of this disease, which are generally accompanied by a high degree of dropsy, are no suitable cases for treatment at any watering place. But if the case is very chronic, and dropsy not far advanced, the Karlsbad or Wildungen waters may afford great relief. Patients who are very weak and anæmic will be benefited by iron waters.

4. Diseases of the Uterine System.

Chronic uterine catarrh, with profuse secretion, is successfully treated by the alkaline muriated or saline waters, the brine baths (*Soolbäder*) being particularly useful, especially for patients of a scrofulous constitution. Complications with enlarged liver or a plethoric constitution require a treatment by Glauber-salt waters, while anæmic patients derive most benefit from the internal and external application of the iron waters. The ascending *douche* is a very powerful remedy in all cases of uterine catarrh. For

Chronic inflammation of the uterus, when combined with great local irritability and general nervous excitability, the waters of Schlangenbad and Landeck are highly praised. If the case is complicated with constipation, the Glaubersalt and saline springs should be used, as they relieve the sexual organs by producing fluid evacuations. Brine and peat baths, which reduce engorgement of the uterus, are eminently beneficial. Anæmic patients of this class should resort to the iron springs, take iron or peat baths, and drink iron water. The chalybeate waters of Elster and Franzensbad enjoy a special reputation for efficacy in such cases.

Irregularities of the menstruation, especially amenorrhœa and dysmenorrhœa, often derive great benefit from the indifferent thermal waters (Schlangenbad), provided that these complaints be not caused by local affections requiring surgical aid. Iron baths are also frequently applied with great success.

Sterility is frequently caused by catarrh of the uterus, anæmia, and excessive nervous irritability. The great reputation of some spas, as, for instance, Ems, and of some iron springs, for a special efficacy in cases of sterility, chiefly depends on the beneficial results obtained there in complaints like the above-named, by the cure of which the cause of sterility is sometimes removed. But when, as is frequently the case, a local obstruction is the cause of the disability, a surgical treatment should be resorted to.

5. Diseases of the Skin.

Some balneologists, especially Braun, who in this this point coincides with Hebra, one of the greatest living authorities on dermatology, deny that any benefit can be derived from mineral waters in the treatment of chronic eruptions of the skin. They denounce the saline baths, which for a long time were considered one of the most efficacious remedies for these evils, as injurious; and the sulphur baths, once praised as the panaceas for all kinds of eruptions, as useless, and not more efficacious than common water baths. Other competent practitioners, particularly the attending physicians at the sulphur and saline springs, claim with great emphasis decided successes obtained by their respective waters.

Chronic eczema, the most frequent of the skin diseases, is contended to be greatly benefited by the use of the sulphur waters of Aachen, Neundorf, &c. Saline baths, though vigorously rejected by some as producing too great an irritation of the skin, are praised by other experienced balneologists (Beneke) as very efficacious, especially those at Nauheim and Kreuznach. For the cure of *impetigo*, sulphur baths are likewise highly recommended (Aachen, Baden, Neundorf, Eilsen). For *psoriasis*, Leuk has a preference, on account of the long-continued immersions.

The indifferent thermal springs (particularly Schlangenbad) are much patronized by patients suffering from a great irritability of the skin, *urticaria* (nettle-rash), *prurigo*, &c.

These waters are also employed with the greatest

advantages for *gunshot wounds, ulcerations* of long standing, either of the skin or the bones, *anchylosis*, &c. Gastein, Ragatz, Wildbad, and especially Teplitz, have been visited by numerous wounded soldiers, after each of the frequent wars, which during the last twenty years have disturbed the peace of Europe.

6. Diseases of the Nervous System.

Hypochondriasis is one of the most frequent complaints treated at the various spas. The regularity in the manner of living, the constant active exercise, and the manifold enjoyments offered at the majority of the spas, exert the most salutary influence upon the mind of hypochondriacs. The local disease which generally is the cause of hypochondriasis, though often of very little importance, is in most cases seated in one of the abdominal organs, and is greatly improved by the use of the proper mineral spring. Sluggishness of the bowels, and a retarded circulation in the abdominal organs being the most frequent symptoms, the cold saline springs are of the greatest benefit to patients of this kind, who cheerfully keep account of the daily evacuations produced by the mineral waters.

If the liver is enlarged and obstinate constipation aggravates the case, the alkaline saline waters (Marienbad, Karlsbad, Tarasp, &c.), are preferable.

Hydropathic treatment is also an unsurpassed remedy for many cases of hypochrondriasis.

Hysteria.—The majority of hysterical patients being anæmic persons with an impaired nutrition, the internal and external application of the iron waters proves highly advantageous. If the anæmia is of little account, but a high degree of nervous irritability prevails, the cool, indifferent thermal springs (Schlangenbad, Johannisbad, &c.), are the proper spas; cases of hysterical paralysis will derive great benefit from the warmer springs of Teplitz, Gastein, &c., or from iron, peat, or saline baths. Favourable results are also sometimes obtained by cautious hydropathic treatment or sea-baths.

Spinal irritation will be benefited by the indifferent thermal springs, iron and sea baths, or by a mild hydropathic treatment.

Neuralgia.—A general rule for the treatment of, neuralgia by mineral waters cannot be established, as the selection of a suitable spring chiefly depends on the cause of the disease. Anæmia very frequently produces neuralgia, especially of the head; cases of this kind are greatly relieved by the use of iron waters. *Sciatica*, if caused by congestions of the abdominal organs, should be treated by saline or alkaline saline waters. Inveterate cases of this obstinate neuralgia are often successfully treated at Teplitz, Wiesbaden, or Aachen. Mountain air has also a very beneficial effect on neuralgic patients.

Paralysis.—Paralysis of the peripheric nerves (i. e., cases where the central organs are not affected) are often caused by rheumatism or by traumatic lesions, or by pressure on the nerves—as, for instance, paralysis in consequence of severe confinements. In such cases splendid results are obtained by the thermal waters of Aachen, Gastein, Teplitz, Ragatz, Wiesbaden, and Wildbad. Peat and mud baths are also very efficacious. In paralysis resulting from inflammation of the brain or spinal cord, if the case is not of too long standing, the warmer indifferent springs, the sulphur spas, the saline waters of Wiesbaden, and peat baths, are recommended. In inveterate, torpid cases, the waters of Kissingen, Nauheim, and Rehme are very useful.

If paralysis is caused by apoplexy, a treatment by mineral waters should not be entered upon unless several months have elapsed after the attack has taken place. The cool indifferent thermal waters should be tried at first; if no favourable results are obtained, the hot indifferent springs, the sulphur or saline baths, should be applied, though with great caution.

Paralysis caused by metallic poisoning derives most benefit from the hot sulphur or indifferent thermal springs. Syphilis is often a cause of paralysis, and the sulphur waters of Aachen have the reputation of being a specific remedy for such cases.

7. Constitutional Diseases.

Scrofula, briefly speaking, is an impure condition of the blood, which renders its victims very prone to disease, especially to consumption, and an easy prey to other acute or chronic diseases. A large part of the human race are more or less tainted with it. Scrofula is chiefly met with in two forms; the one called the *torpid* form is characterized by swelling of the lymphatic glands, particularly those of the neck; the other is called the *erethic* form. Patients of the latter class are slender and delicate, and have a tender skin with transparent veins, and a great irritability of the nervous system. Each form is differently treated, the first form being chiefly benefited by the internal use of the saline springs, the alkaline saline waters, or the *Thassilo* spring of Hall (Austria), and the *Adelheid* spring of Heilbronn (Würtemberg), both containing iodine and bromine. With this internal treatment the external application of the saline waters in the shape of strong brine baths (at Kreuznach, Rehme, Ischl, &c.) should be combined. A sojourn in a high Alpine region also proves highly beneficial.

Scrofulous patients of the second class, i.e. of the erethic form, should try to effect a regeneration of the whole system by country and sea air, warm sea-baths, mild saline baths, proper diet, and a sojourn during the winter at a southern climatic station.

Scrofulous persons who are affected with eruptions on the skin, will derive considerable advantage from the use of the sulphur waters and saline baths.

Rachitis requires a similar treatment. A stay at a sea-side resort and saline baths are highly recommended.

Gout.—The *internal* employment of the alkaline and alkaline saline waters affords the principal curative agent for the treatment of gout. Neuenahr, Bertrich, Ems, and especially Karlsbad, are very efficacious. The cold Glaubersalt springs of Marienbad, Tarasp, &c., also act beneficially, particularly if sluggishness of the bowels, or enlarged and fatty liver, complicate the case. Weak patients will derive benefit from the saline springs of Wiesbaden, Kissingen, &c. If the urinary system is affected, as is often the case in the later stages of gout, the earthy waters of Wildungen or Leuk are preferred.

All these waters prevent the accumulation of lithic acid in the blood, and promote the elimination of the latter by means of the kidneys, the skin, and the alimentary canal. But a proper dietetic regimen is absolutely necessary for the success of the treatment, no matter which spring may be resorted to. Gouty patients should abstain from strong coffee and tea, strong wines and beer, nor should they eat much meat; they should rather confine themselves to a vegetable diet, and indulge in drinking large quantities of water.

The *external* application of mineral waters is of the highest importance, recent exudations in the joints being removed by the energetic use of thermal baths. Old ones will not be resolved.

The most popular spas for gouty patients are, Gastein, Teplitz, Wildbad, Ragatz, Warmbrunn. In cases of long duration, where a great nervous excitability prevails, the cooler indifferent thermal waters, especially those of Schlangenbad, are very useful. The saline baths of Wiesbaden, and the earthy waters of Leuk are likewise very efficacious; sulphur baths are also highly recommended. Gouty exudations and stiffened joints often improve considerably by the application of mud and peat baths.

Rheumatism.—The thermal springs of Teplitz, Gastein, Ragatz, and Warmbrunn have for hundreds of years enjoyed a well-deserved popularity in the cure of rheumatism. The saline waters of Wiesbaden and Baden-Baden, the stronger brine baths of Ischl, Reichenhall, &c., and the thermal saline waters of Nauheim and Rehme, are likewise of great value in removing rheumatic exudations. Chronic rheumatism of the joints is very successfully treated by sulphur, mud, and vapour baths, as practised at Aachen, Burtscheid, and other sulphur spas. The method of protracted baths at Leuk is also of considerable advantage in thickening of the joints. Peat baths are highly praised for weak and irritable patients.

Diabetes is treated at Karlsbad, Neuenahr, and Tarasp, the first of these spas being the most frequented by diabetic patients. The dietetic regimen, which has been sufficiently explained in the third part of this treatise, is of the utmost importance, and a patient who is not willing to submit to it, should never hope to recover.

Metallic poisoning from mercury or lead is benefited by warm mineral baths of whatever kind; but the sulphur springs are the most popular, and patients consider them more powerful than all others.

Syphilis.—Sulphur springs are extensively used in the treatment of this disease, and they are undoubtedly excellent adjuncts to the anti-syphilitic treatment by mercury or iodine. Other thermal waters may produce the same effect, but the sulphur spas have the advantage of an excellent method of treatment, as applied at Aachen and other sulphur springs.

Dr. Beumont (Aachen) claims a particular efficacy of the sulphur waters :—

(1) For patients having already passed through an anti-syphilitic course, if there still is some suspicion

of a latent syphilitic poison. In such cases the treatment by sulphur waters is considered a test for the presence of the disease.

(2) For patients when there is a doubt, whether the symptoms they present are caused by mercury or syphilis, or by any other dyscrasy.

(3) For syphilitic patients suffering from mercurialism or rheumatism. In such cases the sulphur baths are taken as a preparatory course of treatment.

(4) For patients who are under anti-syphilitic treatment. In these cases the sulphur waters materially aid the operation of the specific anti-syphilitic remedies.

Anæmia, caused by hemorrhage and other exhaustive affections, is easily cured by the use of iron waters.

Chlorosis is also successfully treated by iron waters, and a sojourn at one of the Alpine resorts.

> " The book is completed,
> And closed, like the day ;
> And the hand that has written it
> Lays it away."—LONGFELLOW.

APPENDIX.

COMPARATIVE TABLES

OF THE

PRINCIPAL CONSTITUENTS OF THE MINERAL WATERS.

TABLE I.
ALKALINE WATERS.

1. Simple Alkaline Waters.   2. Alkaline Muriated Waters.

Amount of chemical constituents in 1000 parts of water.	Salzbrunn. Oberbrunnen.	Giesshübel. Ottosquelle.	Neuenahr.	Gleichenberg. Constantin-quelle.	Kränchen.	Ems. Kessel-brunnen.	Kaiser-brunnen.
Solids	4·1268	2·1876	2·0646	6·8701	3·5192	3·5515	3·5417
Bicarbonate of soda	2·4240	1·2622	1·0500	3·5545	1·9790	1·9896	1·9920
Chloride of sodium	0·1719	0·0399	0·0907	1·8570	0·9831	1·0313	0·9802
Sulphate of soda	0·4773	0·0489	0·1125	0·0794	0·0335	0·0150	0·0213
Carbonate of magnesia	0·5044	0·2694	0·4373	0·7224	0·2069	0·1824	0·2052
Carbonate of lime	0·4781	0·3618	0·3024	0·5101	0·2161	0·2196	0·2266
Sulphate of potassium	0·0268	0·0676	—	—	0·0367	0·0436	0·0446
Carbonic acid	630·49	1537·7	498·5	1149·75	597·48	553·16	—
Temperature	47°	50°	104°	64°	96°	114°	84°

APPENDIX. 319

3. Alkaline Saline Waters.
(Glaubersalt Waters.)

Amount of chemical constituents in 1000 parts of water.	Karlsbad.			Marienbad.			Franzensbad.	Elster.	Bertrich.	Rohitsch.	Tarasp.
	Sprudel.	Mühlbrunnen.		Ferdinands.	Kreuzbrunnen.		Salzquelle.	Salzquelle.		Tenzelbrunnen.	Luciusquelle.
Solids	5·5168	5·4730		10·6130	11·1073		5·4065	8·3250	1·9013	7·4257	15·7902
Sulphate of soda	2·4053	2·3911		5·0477	4·9531		2·8020	5·2820	0·9209	2·0242	2·1004
Bicarbonate of soda	1·2980	1·2790		1·8228	1·6628		0·9581	1·6849	0·2613	1·0758	5·4579
Chloride of sodium	1·0418	1·0288		2·0047	1·7011		1·1406	0·8276	0·4350	0·0945	3·6739
Carbonate of lime	0·3214	0·3266		0·7839	0·7481		0·2643	0·1819	0·1172	2·2263	2·7539
Carbonate of magnesia	0·1665	0·1613		0·6899	0·6612		0·1567	0·1686	0·0978	1·9704	1·1174
Carbonate of iron	—	—		—	—		0·0125	0·0627	—	—	—
Carbonic acid	104·017	180·304		1127·74	552·61		831·42	986·84	120·09	1129·02	1060
Temperature	162°	132°		78°	52°		50°	48°	89°	50°	44°

TABLE II.
SALINE WATERS.
1. Saline Springs.

Amount of chemical constituents in 1000 parts of water.	Kissingen.		Homburg.		Nauheim.	Rehme.	Pyrmont.	Soden.				Wiesbaden.
	Rakorry.	Pandur.	Elizabeth-brunnen.	Ludwigs-brunnen.	Kur-brunnen.	Bitter-brunnen.	Salz-quelle.	I.	III.	IV.	VI. A.	Koch-brunnen.
Solids	8·5563	7·9960	13·2973	7·0818	18·6828	16·668	10·7006	3·3990	4·7817	16·9259	14·4476	8·2626
Chl. of sodium ...	5·8220	5·5207	9·8609	5·1192	15·4215	12·062	7·0574	2·4255	3·4258	14·2328	13·5549	6·8356
Chl. of potassium	0·2869	0·2414	0·3462	0·2355	0·5270	—	—	0·1366	0·1191	0·6560	0·3295	0·1458
Chl. of magnesium	0·3037	0·2116	0·7288	0·3743	0·7387	0·770	—	—	—	0·1118	—	0·2039
Sulp. of magnesia.	0·5883	0·5977	—	—	—	—	0·9696	—	—	—	—	—
Sulphate of lime...	0·3893	0·3004	0·0168	0·0124	0·0238	3·244	0·8059	—	—	0·0903	0·1280	0·0902
Carbonate of lime.	1·0609	1·0148	1·5106	0·7964	0·7908	0·560	1·6886	0·4593	0·6393	1·3131	0·1920	0·4180
Carbonate of iron.	—	—	—	—	—	—	—	0·0079	0·0118	0·0152	0·0394	—
Carbonic acid	1305·5	1305·5	1407·0	1612·5	9952·2	—	954·0	951·4	1015·5	845·1	1500·0	200·5
Temperature	50°	50°	50°	51°	70°	—	50°	74°	72°	70°	66°	156°

2. Saline Baths.

(a.) Mild Saline Baths.

Amount of chemical constituents in 1000 parts of water.	Wies-baden. Spriegel-quelle.	Baden-Baden. Brüh-quelle.	Baden-Baden. Ur-sprung.	Kreuznach. Elisen-quelle.	Kreuznach. Oranien-quelle.	Cannstadt. Wilhelms-brunn.	Cannstadt. Sprudel.
Chloride of sodium	6·824	2·2266	2·1511	9·494	14·153	2·010	2·044
Chloride of potassium	0·143	0·1729	0·1638	0·126	0·059	—	—
Carbonate of lime	0·415	0·1937	0·1657	—	0·032	1·057	1·067
Solids	8·1	3·0014	2·8767	—	—	4·861	4·808
Carbonic acid	248·5	30·87	2472	—	—	865·6	987·5
Temperature	152°	156°	156°	54°	54°	66°	70°

(b.) Strong Saline Baths (Soolbäder).

Amount of chemical constituents in 1000 parts of water.	Ischl. Ischler Soole (brine.)	Reichen-hall.	Aussee.	Pyrmont.
Chloride of sodium	236·13	224·36	244·5	32·005
Chloride of potassium	—	—	—	1·628
Carbonate of lime	—	0·010	—	—
Solids	245·49	233·0	272·78	40·4
Carbonic acid	—	—	—	373·0
Temperature	—	—	—	—

(c.) Saline Baths with Iodine and Bromine.

Amount of chemical constituents in 1000 parts of water.	Hall. Thassilo-quelle.	Kreuznach. Elisen-quelle.	Kreuznach. Oranien-quelle.	Münster-am-Stein.
Chloride of sodium	12·170	9·494	14·153	7·900
Chloride of potassium	0·039	0·126	0·059	0·174
Carbonate of lime	—	—	0·032	—
Iodide of magnesium	0·0426	0·00039	0·0014	—
Bromide of magnesium	0·0584	0·0399	0·231	—
Carbonate of soda	—	—	—	—
Solids	13·067	11·799	17·638	9·93185
Bromide of soda	—	—	—	0·076
Carbonic acid	120	—	—	—
Temperature	52°	54°	54°	86°

(d.) Saline Baths rich in Carbonic Acid.

	Rehme-Oeynhausen. Thermal salt well.	Nauheim. Grosser Sprudel.	Kissin-gen. Sool-sprudel.	Soden. Soolsprudel, xiv.
Chloride of sodium	30·351	21·8245	10·5540	14·5500
Chloride of potassium	—	0·4974	—	0·5937
Carbonate of lime	1·005	2·3541	1·3046	1·2950
Bromide of magnesium	—	0·0060	—	0·0012
Carbonate of soda	—	—	—	—
Solids	39·5503	26·3539	14·2994	16·8674
Carbonic acid	753·7	712·65	764	756·0
Temperature	89°	89°	64°	86°

Table III.

SULPHUR WATERS.

1. Warm Sulphur Waters.

	Aachen (Aix la Chapelle). Kaiserquelle.	Burtscheid. Victoriabrunnen.	Landeck. Wiesenquelle.	Baden (near Vienna). Ursprung.	Baden (Switzerland).
Chloride of sodium	2·6161	2·7913	0·0072	0·2552	0·3204
Carbonate of soda	0·6449	0·6242	0·0726	0·0937	—
Sulphate of soda ..	0·2836	0·2817	0·0822	0·3013	1·8427
Sulphate of potass.	0·1527	0·1665	—	0·0729	0·1273
Solids	4·0791	4·1245	0·2173	2·1687	3·9700
Temperature	132°	142°	80°	94°	116°

2. Cold Sulphur Waters.

	Nenndorf. Trinkquelle.	Eilsen. Julianenquelle.	Weilbach. Schwefelquelle.	Meinberg. Schwefelquelle.
Chloride of sodium	—	—	0·2712	0·0833
Carbonate of soda	— —	—	0·2874	—
Sulphate of soda	0·564	—	—	0·2356
Sulphate of potass	0·042	—	0·0388	0·0007
Carbonate of lime	0·419	—	0·1816	0·2960
Sulphate of lime	1·007	1·7914	—	0·8337
Total contents	2·636	2·7122	1·0637	1·6927
Temperature	53°	53°	56°	52°—60°
Sulphuretted hydrogen ...	42·31	40·41	5·08	23·1
Carbonic acid	173·03	67·22	262·01	81·1
Nitrogen	20·30	11·69	—	14·1

TABLE IV.
IRON WATERS.

	Bocklet.	Brückenau.	Cudowa.	Driburg.		Elster.		Franzensbad.	
	Stahl-brunnen.	Alte Quelle.	Ober-brunnen.	Wiesen-quelle.	Kaiser-Wilhelmquelle.	Königs-quelle.	Moritz-quelle.	Franzens-quelle.	Stahl-quelle.
Bicarbonate of iron	0·1211	0·0120	0·0271	0·0798	0·0436	0·0840	0·0858	0·0413	0·0781
" " soda	—	—	0·9505	—	—	0·7355	0·2613	0·9544	0·5469
" " lime	0·6759	0·2276	0·5531	1·5148	0·6122	0·2552	0·1520	0·3375	0·1992
" " magnesia	0·6813	0·0207	0·1879	0·0867	0·6194	0·1194	0·1093	0·1329	0·0534
Chloride of sodium	0·8541	—	0·0914	0·1681	0·0731	1·4750	0·6647	1·2018	0·6119
Sulphate of soda	0·3309	0·0107	0·5452	0·2447	0·4616	2·0866	0·9547	3·1901	1·6164
Total constituents	3·6875	0·4448	2·5047	2·1386	3·5520	4·9009	2·2824	5·9352	3·1874
Carbonic acid	1505·01	1298·0	1251·38	1165·2	1325	1310·92	1266·12	1467·68	1528·96
Temperature	50°	49°	52°	52°	49°	50°	49°	50°	54°

	Homburg.	St. Moritz.	Pyrmont.			Reinerz.		Schwalbach.		
	Stahl-brunnen.	Alte Quelle.	Stahl-brunnen.	Helenen-brunnen.	Brodel-brunnen.	Lave-quelle.	Ulriken-quelle.	Stahl-brunnen.	Wein-brunnen.	Neu-brunnen.
Bicarbonate of iron	0·0984	0·0330	0·0770	0·0966	0·0743	0·0519	0·0216	0·0837	0·0578	0·0771
" " soda	—	0·2773	—	—	—	0·7860	0·3849	0·0206	0·2453	0·0235
" " lime	1·0403	1·2269	1·0468	1·0037	1·2469	1·1800	0·5940	0·2213	0·5721	0·2527
" " magnesia	0·0935	0·1970	0·0802	0·0760	0·0127	0·3565	0·1447	0·2122	0·0651	0·2238
Chloride of sodium	5·8631	0·0437	0·1588	0·1743	0·1810	0·0157	—	0·0067	0·0086	0·0062
Sulphate of soda	—	0·3074	—	—	0·0435	—	—	0·0079	0·0061	0·0094
Total constituents	8·2235	2·1497	2·7130	2·8584	3·1013	2·5449	1·3056	0·6058	1·5582	0·6685
Carbonic acid	1082·93	1230·01	1271·05	1305·5	1323·72	1097·02	1110·88	1570·9	1425·0	1429·6
Temperature	52°	42°	54°	55°	55°	64°	54°	46°–50°	46°–50°	48°

TABLE V.
EARTHY WATERS.

Amount of chemical constituents in 1000 parts.	Lippspringe. Arminius-quelle.	Inselbad. Ottilien-quelle.	Leuk. Lorenz-quelle.	Helenen-quelle.	Wildungen. Georg-Vic-torquelle.	Königs-quelle.	Bormio.
Sulphate of lime	0·824	0·085	1·520	—	—	—	0·4863
Sulphate of soda	0·846	—	0·050	0·013	0·068	0·0127	0·0604
Carbonate of lime	0·416	0·309	0·005	0·881	0·494	0·8520	0·1735
Bicarbonate of lime	0·602	0·453	0·007	1·269	0·712	1·2268	—
Carbonate of magnesia	0·034	0·036	0·009	0·895	0·351	0·7181	—
Bicarbonate of magnesia	0·051	0·056	0·014	1·363	0·535	1·0943	—
Carbonate of iron	0·014	0·0002	0·010	0·013	0·015	0·0268	0·0025
Bicarbonate of iron	0·019	0·0004	0·013	0·018	0·021	0·0369	—
Chloride of sodium	0·033	0·771	—	1·043	0·007	1·3079	0·0112
Bicarbonate of soda	—	—	—	0·845	0·064	0·0951	—
Total constituents	2·404	1·446	1·989	4·616	1·443	3·8698	1·0261
Carbonic acid in 1000 c.c. parts of water	—	461·04	2·389	1351·2	1322·2	—	24·56
Temperature	70°	64°	124°	52°	50°	52°	102°
The gas emanating from the spring contains:—							
Carbonic acid	149·0	—	—	—	—	—	—
Nitrogen	824·4	—	—	—	—	—	—
Oxygen	26·6	—	—	—	—	—	—

Table VI.

INDIFFERENT THERMAL WATERS.

	Elevation.	Temperature of the thermal water.
	Feet.	Deg. Fahr.
Gastein	3400	96—118
Johannisbad	1940	86
Neuhaus	1200	95
Ragatz-Pfäffers	1566—2050	94—99
Römerbad	731	97—102
Schlangenbad	925	82—92
Teplitz	715	86—118
Tobelbad	1072	87
Tüffer	700	95—102
Warmbrunn	1198	96—108
Wildbad	1300	93—98
Villach	1500	84

COIN TABLE.

Countries.	Coin.	Mark.	Pfennige.	Gulden (florin.)	Kreuzer.	Franc.	Centimes.	Shillings.	Pence.	Dollar.	Cents.
Germany	1 mark = 100 pfernige	1	—	—	50	1	25	1	—	—	24
Austria	1 gulden = 100 kreuzer	2	—	1	—	2	50	2	—	—	47
France / Switzerland	1 franc = 100 centimes	—	80	—	40	1	—	—	9½	—	19
England	1 pound = 20 shillings (1 shilling = 12 pence)	20	—	10	—	25	—	20	—	4	80
U. S. of America	1 dollar = 100 cents	4	16	2	12	5	25	4	2	1	—

INDEX OF WATERING PLACES AND HEALTH RESORTS.

AACHEN (Aix-la-Chapelle), 75, 224.
Adelheidsquelle, 312.
Ajaccio, 269.
Albisbrunn, 299.
Alveneu, 167, 224.
Arco, 276.
Aussee, 151, 214, 282.

BADEN-BADEN, 102, 202, 210.
Baden (Austria), 146, 226.
Baden (Switzerland), 162, 226.
Bertrich, 79, 197.
Bocklet, 99, 235.
Borkum, 285.
Bormio, 169, 243.
Botzen, 276.
Brestenberg, 299.
Brückenau, 100, 235.
Burtscheid, 225.

CAIRO, 268.
Cannstadt, 110, 202, 210.
Catania, 269.
Cudowa, 117, 235.

DAVOS, 281.
Dietenmühle, 299.
Driburg, 74, 236.
Dürkheim, 298.

EILSEN, 68, 223.
Elster, 144, 196, 236.
Ems, 88, 182.
Eggenberg, 300.

FRANZENSBAD, 142, 236, 304.

GASTEIN, 152, 251.
Geisshübel, 182.
Gleichenberg, 155, 183.
Görbersdorf, 278.
Godesberg, 299.
Gräfenberg, 300.
Gries, 276.

HALL, 148, 212, 298, 312.
Heligoland, 285.
Homburg, 93, 202, 237.
Hyères, 270.

INNICHEN, 161.
Inselbad, 74, 242.
Ischl, 149, 213.

JOHANNISBAD, 145, 251.

KALTENLEUTGEBEN, 300.
Karlsbad, 121, 184.
Kissengen, 97, 202, 214.

INDEX OF WATERING PLACES, ETC.

Königsbrunn, 300.
Kreuth, 113, 213, 298.
Kreuznach, 79, 211.

LANDECK, 116, 225.
Leuk, 171, 243.
Le Prese, 168, 224, 298.
Lippspringe, 73, 241.

MADEIRA, 267.
Marienbad, 139, 195.
Marienberg, 299.
Meinberg, 72, 223.
Mentone, 272.
Meran, 275, 298.
Montreux, 276.
Mühlbad, 299.
Münster-am-Stein, 82, 212.

NAUHEIM, 96, 216.
Naples, 274.
Neundorf, 222.
Nerothal, 299.
Neuenahr, 78, 182.
Nice, 271.
Norderney, 285.

OBERMAIS, 300.
Ostend, 284.

PALERMO, 268.
Priessnitzthal, 300.
Pyrmont, 70, 215, 237.

RAGATZ-PFÄFFERS, 164, 252.

Rehme-Oeynhausen, 215.
Reichenhall, 111, 213.
Reinerz, 117, 238.
Römerbad, 159, 252.
Rohitsch, 157, 196.
Rome, 274.

SALZBRUNN (Obersalzbrunn), 114, 182.
Scheveningen, 284.
Schlangenbad, 87, 250.
Schwalbach (Langenschwalbach), 85, 238.
Schönbrunn, 299.
Schönegg, 299.
Schweizermühle, 300.
Soden, 92, 217.
St. Moritz, 167, 237.
San Remo, 273.
Sylt, 284.

TARASP, 170, 195.
Teplitz, 135, 251.
Tobelbad, 156, 251.
Tüffer, 158, 252.

VENICE, 274.
Vevey, 276.
Villach, 160, 251.
Vöslau, 148.

WARMBRUNN, 115, 252.
Weilbach, 91, 223.
Wiesbaden, 82, 210.
Wildbad, 108, 252.
Wildungen, 101, 242.

GENERAL INDEX.

ABSORPTION, 59.
Aftercure, 49.
After-effects, 50.
Air, change of, 253.
——, city, 60.
——, country, 61.
——, mountain, 62.
——, sea, 63.
Anæmia, 230, 299, 315.
Atony of the skin, 209, 216.

BADFRIESEL, 38.
Bath-course, duration of, 40.
—— life, 23.
—— physicians, 13.
——, selection of, 7.
Bathing, time for, 34.
Baths, number of common, 21.
——, herb, 290.
——, indifferent, 57, 245.
——, iron, 227.
——, mud, 288.
——, peat, 287.
——, pine-needle, 289.
——, sand, 288.
——, saline, 198.
Bazaars, 20.
Bitters, 298.
Brines, 207.
Bladder, catarrh of the, 241, 305.

Bright's disease, 306.
Brunnenfieber, 40.

CARBONIC ACID, 58, 198, 217, 231.
Catarrh, bronchial, 177, 196, 202, 305.
————, intestinal, 303.
————, larynx, 293, 304.
————, stomach, 178, 189, 196, 302.
Chlorosis, 315.
Clothing, 26.
Coffee-gardens, 26.
Coin, 11.
Company, 33.
Constipation, 190, 201, 304.
Consumption, 183, 253, 266, 292, 294.
Course, preparatory, 49.

DANCING, 32.
Diabetes, 180, 191, 314.
Diet, 42, 265.
Drinking, time for, 24.
Dyspepsia, 178, 189, 302.

EXERCISE, active, 25, 29.
————, mental, 31.

FRUIT, 46.

Z

GALLSTONES, 181, 190, 304.
Germs, 61.
Glaubersalt, 179.
Gout, 181, 191, 209, 243, 312.
Grape-cure, 295.
Gravel, 181, 191, 241, 306.

HEMORRHOIDS, 303.
Heights, Alpine, 256.
Herb juices, 298.
Hotels, 117, 118.
Hydrogen, sulphuretted, 219, 223.
Hypochondriasis, 309.
Hysteria, 309.
Hydropathy, 298.

IRON, internal use of, 229.
———, external use of, 233.
Irritation, spinal, 310.

JAUNDICE, 304.

KURTAXF, 21.
Kumys, 294.

LIME, 239.
Liver, enlargement of the, 190, 196, 303.
Lodgings, 13.

MILK-CURE, 290.
Morality, 20.
Mutterlauge, 208.

NERVE-BATHS, 247.
Neuralgia, 250, 310.

OBESITY, 191, 195, 196, 303, 304.

PARALYSIS, 215, 222, 225, 310.
Passport, 12.
Poisoning, metallic, 223, 225, 226, 244, 314.

Promenading, 25.

RACHITIS, 240, 312.
Regions, elevated, 277.
Resorts, climatic, 253.
———, southern, 267.
———, seaside, 283.
Review, topographical, 64.
Rheumatism, 209, 216, 243, 251, 313.
Routes to the Continent, 9.

SALT, common, 198.
Sanitarium, 278.
Sciatica, 288, 310.
Scrofula, 201, 204, 208, 311.
Sea-baths, 283.
Skin diseases, 225, 243, 308.
Sleep, 29.
Society, 16.
Soda, 177.
Sommerfrischen, 282.
Spleen, enlargement, 190, 304.
Sterility, 183, 307.
Stomach ulcerations, 178, 189, 303.
Sulphur, 218.
Syphilis, 314.

TABLES-D'HÔTE, 27.
Theatre, 32.
Travelling, after the bath-cure, 51.
————, benefit of, 2.
————, time for, 7.

UTERUS, catarrh, 306.
————, inflammation, 307.
————, tumours, 209.

WATER, cold, 55.
———, warm, 55.
———, external use, 56.
———, internal use, 53.

Water, mineral, 55.
Waters, alkaline, 176.
——, alkaline muriated, 182.
——, alkaline saline, 184.
——, bottled, 4.
——, classification of, 175.
——, earthy, 239.
——, indifferent thermal, 245.
——, iron, 227.
——, saline, 198.
——, sulphur, 218.

Watering places,—introductory remarks, 64.
——————— of Germany, 67.
——————— Austria, 119.
——————— Switzerland, 162
———————, general features of, 15.

WHEY, 292.
Wildbäder, 245.
Wounds, gunshot, 249, 309.

THE END.

GILBERT AND RIVINGTON, PRINTERS, ST. JOHN'S SQUARE, LONDON.

www.ingramcontent.com/pod-product-compliance
Lightning Source LLC
Chambersburg PA
CBHW020242240426
43672CB00006B/610